T0229120

African Skin and Hair Disorders

Editor

NONHLANHLA P. KHUMALO

DERMATOLOGIC CLINICS

www.derm.theclinics.com

Consulting Editor
BRUCE H. THIERS

April 2014 • Volume 32 • Number 2

ELSEVIER

1600 John F. Kennedy Boulevard ● Suite 1800 ● Philadelphia, Pennsylvania, 19103-2899

http://www.theclinics.com

DERMATOLOGIC CLINICS Volume 32, Number 2
April 2014 ISSN 0733-8635, ISBN-13: 978-0-323-28997-9

Editor: Joanne Husovski
Developmental Editor: Susan Showalter

Dermatologic Clinics (ISSN 0733-8635) is published quarterly by Elsevier Inc., 360 Park Avenue South, New York, NY 10010-1710. Months of publication are January, April, July, and October. Business and editorial offices: 1600 John F. Kennedy Blvd., Suite 1800, Philadelphia, PA 19103-2899. Customer service office: 11830 Westline Drive, St. Louis, MO 63146. Periodicals postage paid at New York, NY, and additional mailing offices. Subscription prices are USD 365.00 per year for US individuals, USD 559.00 per year for US institutions, USD 425.00 per year for Canadian individuals, USD 681.00 per year for Canadian institutions, USD 495.00 per year for international individuals, USD 681.00 per year for international institutions, USD 165.00 per year for US students/residents, and USD 240.00 per year for Canadian and international students/residents. International air speed delivery is included in all *Clinics* subscription prices. All prices are subject to change without notice. **POSTMASTER:** Send address changes to *Dermatologic Clinics*, Elsevier Health Sciences Division, Subscription Customer Service, 3251 Riverport Lane, Maryland Heights, MO 63043. **Customer Service: 1-800-654-2452 (U.S. and Canada); 314-447-8871 (outside U.S. and Canada). Fax: 314-447-8029. E-mail: journalscustomerservice-usa@elsevier.com (for print support); journalsonlinesupport-usa@elsevier.com (for online support).**

Reprints. For copies of 100 or more, of articles in this publication, please contact the Commercial Reprints Department, Elsevier Inc., 360 Park Avenue South, New York, New York 10010-1710. Tel.: 212-633-3874; Fax: 212-633-3820; E-mail: reprints@elsevier.com.

The *Dermatologic Clinics* is covered in *MEDLINE/PubMed (Index Medicus)*, *Current Contents/Clinical Medicine, Excerpta Medica, Chemical Abstracts,* and *ISI/BIOMED.*

Contributors

CONSULTING EDITOR

BRUCE H. THIERS, MD
Professor and Chairman, Department of
Dermatology and Dermatologic Surgery,
Medical University of South Carolina,
Charleston, South Carolina

EDITOR

**NONHLANHLA P. KHUMALO, MBChB,
FCDerm (SA), PhD**
Professor, Head, Division of Dermatology,
Groote Schuur Hospital, University of Cape
Town, Cape Town, Western Province,
South Africa

AUTHORS

ANDREW ALEXIS, MD, MPH
Associate Professor, Mount Sinai School of
Medicine, Department of Dermatology,
Director, Skin of Color Center,
St. Luke's-Roosevelt Hospital, Mount Sinai
Heath System, New York,
New York

ARDESHIR BAYAT, MBBS, MRCS, PhD
Plastic and Reconstructive Surgery
Research, Manchester Institute of
Biotechnology, University of Manchester;
Plastic and Reconstructive Surgery
Research, Faculty of Medical and Human
Sciences, Institute of Inflammation and
Repair, University Hospital of South
Manchester NHS Foundation Trust,
Manchester Academic Health Science
Centre, University of Manchester,
Manchester, United Kingdom

ACHILÉA BITTENCOURT, MD
Laboratory Service, Complexo Hospitalar
Universita'rio Prof Edgars Santos, University
of Bahia, Salvador, Bahia, Brazil

VALERIE D. CALLENDER, MD, FAAD
Associate Professor of Dermatology, Howard
University College of Medicine, Washington,
DC; Medical Director, Callender Dermatology &
Cosmetic Center, Glenn Dale, Maryland

GEORGE CHAPLIN, MSc
Senior Research Associate, Departments of
Anthropology and Geography, The Pennsylvania
State University, University Park, Pennsylvania

ZOE DIANA DRAELOS, MD
Consulting Professor, Department of
Dermatology, Duke University School of
Medicine, Durham, North Carolina

REBAT M. HALDER, MD
Professor and Chairman, Department of
Dermatology, Howard University College of
Medicine, Washington, DC

CANDRICE R. HEATH, MD
Department of Dermatology, Resident
Physician, St. Luke's-Roosevelt Hospital,
Mount Sinai Health System, New York,
New York

CAROL HLELA, PhD, MD
Division of Dermatology, Red Cross War
Memorial Children's Hospital, University of
Cape Town, Rondebosch, Cape Town,
Western Cape, South Africa

NINA G. JABLONSKI, PhD
Distinguished Professor of Anthropology,
Department of Anthropology, The Pennsylvania
State University, University Park, Pennsylvania

**MAHLATSE KGOKOLO, BPharm, MBChB,
MMed, FCDerm(SA)**
Department of Dermatology University of Pretoria,
Steve Biko Hospital, Pretoria, South Africa

**NONHLANHLA P. KHUMALO, MBChB,
FCDerm (SA), PhD**
Professor, Head, Division of Dermatology, Groote
Schuur Hospital, University of Cape Town, Cape
Town, Western Province, South Africa

**RANNAKOE J. LEHLOENYA, BSc, MBChB,
FCDerm(SA)**
Division of Dermatology, Department of
Medicine, University of Cape Town, Cape
Town, South Africa

AMY MCMICHAEL, MD
Professor and Chair, Department of
Dermatology, Wake Forest Baptist Health,
Winston-Salem, North Carolina

PARADI MIRMIRANI, MD
Department of Dermatology, The Permanente
Medical Group, Vallejo, California; Department
of Dermatology, University of California, San
Francisco, California; Department of
Dermatology, Case Western Reserve
University, Cleveland, Ohio

VANESSA E. MOLINAR, BA
Paul L. Foster School of Medicine, Texas Tech
University Health Sciences Center, El Paso, Texas

**MOJAKGOMO HENDRICK MOTSWALEDI,
MBChB, MMED(Derm), FCDerm(SA)**
Department of Dermatology, University of
Limpopo (Medunsa Campus), Pretoria,
South Africa

TEMITAYO A. OGUNLEYE, MD
Assistant Professor, Department of
Dermatology, Perelman Center for Advanced
Medicine, University of Pennsylvania,
Philadelphia, Pennsylvania

ELISE A. OLSEN, MD
Professor of Dermatology and Medicine,
Director, Department of Dermatology, Hair
Disorders Research and Treatment Center,
Duke University Medical Center, Durham,
North Carolina

AMIT G. PANDYA, MD
Professor, Department of Dermatology,
University of Texas Southwestern Medical
Center, Dallas, Texas

NICOLE E. ROGERS, MD, FAAD
Assistant Clinical Professor, Department of
Dermatology, Tulane University School of
Medicine, New Orleans; Medical Director,
Hair Restoration of the South, Metairie,
Louisiana

SUSAN C. TAYLOR, MD
Assistant Clinical Professor of Dermatology,
College of Physicians and Surgeons, Columbia
University Medical Center, New York,
New York; Society Hill Dermatology,
Philadelphia, Pennsylvania

ANTONELLA TOSTI, MD
Department of Dermatology and Cutaneous
Surgery, University of Miami Miller School of
Medicine, Miami, Florida

SARA UD-DIN, MSc
Plastic and Reconstructive Surgery Research,
Manchester Institute of Biotechnology,
University of Manchester; Plastic and
Reconstructive Surgery Research, Faculty
of Medical and Human Sciences, Institute of
Inflammation and Repair, University Hospital of
South Manchester NHS Foundation Trust,
Manchester Academic Health Science Centre,
University of Manchester, Manchester,
United Kingdom

**WILLIE VISSER, MBChB, MFamMed,
MMED(Derm)**
Division of Dermatology, Department of
Medicine, University of Stellenbosch,
Cape Town, South Africa

NATALIE C. YIN, MD
Department of Dermatology and Cutaneous
Surgery, University of Miami Miller School of
Medicine, Miami, Florida

Contents

Our species, *Homo sapiens*, evolved in Africa, and humanity's highest levels of genetic diversity are maintained there today. Underlying genetic diversity combined with the great range of solar regimes and climatic conditions found in Africa has contributed to a wide range of human integumentary phenotypes within the continent. Millions of Africans have moved, voluntarily and involuntarily, to other continents in the past 2000 years, and the range of integumentary phenotypes among admixed African diaspora populations is enormous. In this contribution, we do not catalog this variation, but provide basic evolutionary background as to how it developed in the first place.

Facial hyperpigmentation is common and challenging to treat in darker-skinned populations. A Medline literature search of articles published up to October 2013 reporting the objective assessment of and/or treatment for melasma, postinflammatory hyperpigmentation, dermatosis papulosa nigra, lichen planus pigmentosus, and erythema dyschromicum perstans was reviewed. Objective assessment was only reported for melasma and postinflammatory hyperpigmentation. Furthermore, randomized controlled trial evidence was only reported for melasma. Although progress has been made, there is a need to develop more objective outcome measures and effective treatments for hyperpigmentation.

Cosmeceuticals are understood to be active cosmetics that are sold over-the-counter, but have profound effects on skin appearance and functioning. This term has no legal meaning in the United States, because only cosmetics and pharmaceuticals are recognized by regulatory bodies. Cosmeceuticals are carefully developed and tested by the cosmetics industry to deliver consumer-recognizable benefits, with an excellent safety profile. Persons use these products worldwide, including those of African descent, for improvement of skin tone. This article discusses the issues surrounding cosmeceutical use by persons of African descent.

Trichoscopy facilitates the diagnosis of various hair and scalp disorders and is often useful in predicting the disease course. However, to date, few studies describe the dermoscopic findings unique to Afro-textured hair. This article reviews what is currently known regarding trichoscopy and discusses its usefulness in this population.

Traction alopecia (TA) affects up to 32% of women and 22% of high school girls with Afro-textured hair but can start in the preschool years. Traction induces inflammation and follicle damage. The risk of TA increases with symptomatic traction and combined hairstyles. To influence the practice of hairdressers and at risk individuals and help narrow the knowledge, attitudes, and practices (KAP) gap, scientific data should be translated into simple messages like "tolerate pain from a hairstyle and risk hair loss" and "no braids or weaves on relaxed hair". With appropriate education and public awareness, TA could potentially be eradicated.

Although the biochemical composition of hair is similar among racial and ethnic groups, the hair structure between them varies, and individuals with curly hair pose specific challenges and special considerations when a surgical option for alopecia is considered. Hair restoration in this population should therefore be approached with knowledge on the clinical characteristics of curly hair, hair grooming techniques that may influence the management, unique indications for the procedure, surgical instrumentation used, and the complications that may arise.

Central centrifugal cicatricial alopecia is an inflammatory type of central scalp hair loss seen primarily in women of African descent. The prevalence is unknown, but may vary from 2.7% to 5.7% and increases with age. This review outlines the history and current beliefs and identifies clues for future research for this enigmatic condition. Despite that the cause of central centrifugal cicatricial alopecia is unknown, research is ongoing. The role of cytokeratins, androgens, genetics, and various possible sources of chronic inflammation in disease pathogenesis remain to be elucidated.

Pseudofolliculitis barbae and folliculitis keloidalis nuchae are chronic follicular disorders disproportionately affecting men of African ancestry. This article explores the etiology, pathogenesis, treatment, and prevention strategies of these conditions. Effective treatment and prevention of these disorders involves pharmacologic and procedural interventions as well as behavioral modifications.

This article presents an overview of the literature regarding treatments for keloid disease, hypertrophic scars, and striae distensae in dark pigmented skin. Striae, keloid, and hypertrophic scarring present a challenging problem for both the clinician and patient. No single therapy is advocated for hypertrophic scars, keloid scars, or striae distensae. New therapies have shown promise in the treatment of hypertrophic and keloid scars, and in patients with dark pigmented skin. This article provides guidance on the assessment and determination of patients' suitability for certain treatment options, as well as advice on the follow-up of patients affected with problematic scarring and striae.

HIV and AIDS patients often suffer from various skin infections of viral, bacterial, and fungal origin. In addition, parasitic infestations are prevalent. Common inflammatory dermatoses include seborrheic dermatitis, psoriasis, photodermatitis, and pruritic papular eruptions. This article discusses some of these conditions with an emphasis on clinical presentation. In patients with pigmented skin, diagnosis maybe challenging and complicated by dyspigmentation.

Sub-Saharan Africa is the epicenter of the HIV pandemic and HIV-infected people are more susceptible to inflammatory dermatoses, infections, and drug eruptions. Many of the drugs used for HIV-associated opportunistic infections are associated with a higher incidence of drug-related toxicities and drug interactions. This article discusses the epidemiology, pharmacogenetics, and clinical features of idiosyncratic drug reactions in HIV-infected Africans. Special considerations in this population, including immune reconstitution inflammatory syndrome, multiple drug hypersensitivity syndrome, drug reactions in pregnancy, drug rechallenge in lichenoid drug eruptions, and anxiety/depression after cutaneous adverse drug reactions, are also briefly discussed.

Infective dermatitis associated with human T-cell lymphotropic virus type 1 (HTLV-1) (IDH) is a chronic dermatitis that has been observed in a variable proportion of HTLV-1–infected children. IDH may serve as an early clinical marker for HTLV-1 infection and an indicator of increased risk for developing other HTLV-1–associated conditions. Factors that lead only some infected children to develop IDH are poorly understood. The variable clinical presentation of IDH, in particular its chronicity, the morphology and distribution of the lesions, and its clinical resemblance to other cutaneous inflammatory conditions, make it necessary to distinguish it from other common dermatoses.

DERMATOLOGIC CLINICS

FORTHCOMING ISSUES

July 2014
Hyperhidrosis
David Pariser, *Editor*

October 2014
Photodermatology
Henry Lim and So Yeon Paek, *Editors*

RECENT ISSUES

January 2014
Cosmetic Dermatology
Neil S. Sadick and Nils Krueger, *Editors*

October 2013
Dermoscopy
Giuseppe Argenziano, Iris Zalaudek, and
Jason Giacomel, *Editors*

April 2013
Pediatric Dermatology
Moise L. Levy, *Editor*

January 2013
**Hair Disorders: Current Concepts in
Pathophysiology, Diagnosis, and
Management**
Jerry Shapiro, *Editor*

RELATED INTEREST

**Structural and functional differences in barrier properties of African American,
Caucasian and East Asian skin**
Neelam Muizzuddin, Lieveke Hellemans, Luc Van Overloop, et al.
Journal of Dermatological Science, August 2010, Volume 59, Issue 2, pages 123–128
http://www.sciencedirect.com/science/journal/09231811
http://www.jdsjournal.com/

Preface
Beyond "Ethnicity" in Dermatology

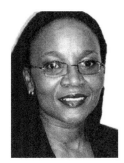

Nonhlanhla P. Khumalo, MBChB, FCDerm, PhD
Editor

People of African ancestry have in common darker hues of skin color and tightly curly hair. These phenotypic features were used as surrogates for "race." More recently, "ethnicity" has appeared with increasing frequency in scientific literature, used together with or as a substitute for race to show signicant[1–5] and insignificant differences between groups.[6–8] Relative poverty and related diseases result largely from historical racial segregation. Studies should, but do not always, control for obvious confounders such as education and social class before inferring causal associations between disease and ethnicity.[9]

Ethnicity has been defined as "a complex multidimensional construct reflecting the confluence of biological factors and geographic origins, culture, economic, political, and legal factors, as well as racism."[10] A useful, simple definition is: "in its most elemental form, ethnicity is an expression of language, culture, social mores and folklore, while race is determined by external features— the most important of which are skin color ... and hair texture."[11] This understanding may have contributed to the move away from the designation: "Black American" to "African American." Ethnicity embodies cultural practices and dietary preferences that may influence disease predilection. However, unlike gender, the use of ethnicity in scientific discourse is problematic as its effect on disease is difficult to measure. With the exception of remote societies, ethnicity is often difficult to categorize, particularly in cities with large admixture.[12] A tangible danger of ethnic profiling is when effective treatment is denied patients because it is deemed ineffective in their group.[13,14] A contrary argument is that abandoning ethnic categories could hide disparities in health care delivery.[15]

The influence of geography (climate, etc) on human variation is worth considering. The relationship between sun exposure and skin cancer is well established. However, sun-induced skin cancers predominantly occur in adults after the reproductive years and are thus unlikely to have exerted an evolutionary force for skin color variation. In this issue of *Dermatologic Clinics*, we are privileged to share the contribution by Jablonski and Chaplin, which elucidates the phenotypic variation within the African continent. They also proposed the most plausible hypothesis for the evolution of skin color.[16,17] They suggested that skin color may have evolved because of the need to balance requirements for vitamin D synthesis versus protection against ultraviolet folate photolysis. Simply put, as humans migrated out of Africa, because of limited sunlight, those with dark skin were unable absorb enough ultraviolet light to synthesize adequate vitamin D (or efficiently absorb calcium for strong bones), were more likely to give birth to children with rickets who were less likely to successfully carry a fetus to term, and were thus selected out of the genetic pool. On the other hand, very pale skin close to the equator is prone to ultraviolet photolysis and folate deficiency. Folate is needed by rapidly dividing cells and deficiency in pregnancy increases the risk of neurologic deformities (eg, anencephaly, spina

Dermatol Clin 32 (2014) ix–xii
http://dx.doi.org/10.1016/j.det.2014.01.001
0733-8635/14/$ – see front matter © 2014 Published by Elsevier Inc.

bifida), which are incompatible with a healthy life and successful reproduction (**Fig. 1**).

The current hypothesis for the evolution of hair curl suggests that tighter curls are better for hot environments. While there is a high correlation of skin color to solar strength worldwide,[13] this may not be the case with hair curl. For example, people in the South of India are as dark as or even darker than most Southern Africans yet have straight hair compared with tightly curly hair. This apparent discordance of skin color and hair curl warrants scientific scrutiny that may advance a new hypothesis for the evolution of hair curl.

Skin color and hair texture are variables that do confer susceptibility to dermatologic disease, as is the case in folliculitis keloidalis and pseudofolliculitis barbae so well discussed by Alexis, Heath, and Halder in this issue. The contribution by Ud-Din and Bayat takes us into the next generation of molecular mechanisms and future potential targeted treatments for keloids, hypertrophic scars, and striae. National regulatory bodies do not recognize cosmeceuticals or "cosmetics with drug-like efficacy." However, because of various skin-benefit claims, their popularity is increasing in all populations. Draelos's article is informative, as cosmeceuticals may confound dermatologic presentations and treatment effects. Taylor, Padya, and Molinar discuss the objective assessment and management of the prevalent problem of facial hyperpigmentation. The widely used Fitzpatrick's classification depends on historic responses to sun exposure and is thus subjective. The use of validated cards with color shades such as the Taylor hyperpigmentation scale seems useful. Colorimetric measurements may be more objective, but no single tool has received universal acceptance.

Until recently, hair curl was classified racially—African, Caucasian, and Asian. Variation within groups becomes magnified when one considers that "Caucasian" hair can range from tightly curly to ultra-straight. The recently published quantitative classification of human hair uses 3 geometric measurements to classify human hair into 8 types.[18] Most Afro-textured hair falls into types 5 through 8. If validated, this classification could help measure the influence of texture on hairstyle choice and alopecia. Mirmira and coauthor present potentially achievable goals. It is not common in medicine that we have, as in traction alopecia (TA), study data that can easily be translated for disease prevention. The challenge is how to bridge the *kap-gap* (ie, the gap between knowledge, attitudes, and practice). Unlike TA, unconquered frontiers include the commonest form of scarring alopecia comprehensively discussed by Ogunleye, McMichael and Olsen. The other is hair restoration–Rogers and Callender are pioneers because many hair transplantation centres do not offer the procedure to patients with tightly curly afro-textured hair. Yin and Tosti demonstrate how dermoscopy complements clinical examination; how it can reduce the need for scalp biopsies and guide the choice of biopsy site.

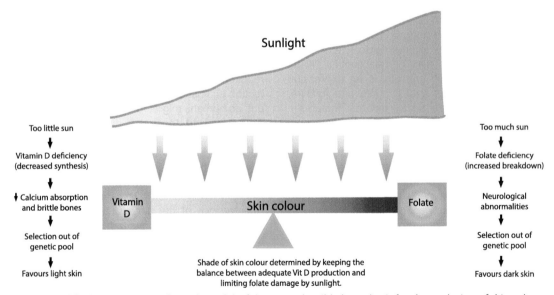

Fig. 1. Simplified representation (N.P. Khumalo) of the most plausible hypothesis for the evolution of skin color; a seesaw balance of 2 factors. Skin color varies globally, evolved to be darker (melanin-rich) in hotter environments to protect against sun-induced folate breakdown, and became paler in cold climates to maximize vitamin D synthesis.

The title of this issue of *Dermatologic Clinics* also infers geography; sub-Saharan Africa has the highest burden of the human immunodeficiency virus (HIV). Motswaledi and Visser, in their contribution on infective and inflammatory disorders in HIV, illustrate dramatic postinflammatory dyspigmentation that often masks the diagnosis and complicates management of common dermatoses. Although antiretrovirals have dramatically improved mortality, the colliding epidemics of tuberculosis and HIV have contributed to an exponential rise in severe adverse drug reactions and exaggerated clinical presentations as eloquently demonstrated by Lehloenya and Kgokolo.

The little known human T-cell leucotropic virus (HTLV-1)-associated dermatitis discussed by Hlela and Bittencourt has been included in this issue of *Dermatologic Clinics* for various reasons. First, HTLV1 is a retrovirus with some similarities to HIV. Second, and important for dermatologists, the infection is associated with a childhood chronic dermatitis that may be mistaken for seborrheic (and atopic) dermatitis. Finally, HTLV1-associated dermatitis in childhood may precede hemopoietic malignancy and disabling neurologic disease in adulthood.

Finally, this issue of *Dermatologic Clinics* focuses on disorders that predominately affect people of African ancestry mostly because of their skin color, hair form, or geographic origin. Several overlapping terms are worth considering:

1. "Phenotype" is an important disease determinant in dermatology (skin color and skin cancer, hair texture and specific alopecias).
2. "Race" is not the same as phenotype or ethnicity and its use should be discarded.
3. "Ethnic skin/hair" is nonspecific and could mean any population subgroup (eg, Greek, Chinese, or fair-skinned Scandinavians).
4. "Ethnicity" is not the same as phenotype (eg, Africans may look similar but be different in every other way—African Muslims are culturally closer to Arabs than sub-Saharan Africans).
5. Ethnicity is difficult to categorize or measure its effect in scientific studies. However, it is important to include where relevant to measure social justice and fairness.

As a result of population migration, skin color and specific genetic susceptibility may correlate.[19] However, variability within groups and admixture make the use of skin color as a general marker of disease predilection unscientific. Skin color and hair texture do influence specific dermatologic disease, but unlike ethnicity, they are amenable to measurement. As dermatologists and scientists, the utopia would be for us to disabuse our discipline of all reference to race and, yes, even ethnicity. Various attempts have been made to objectively classify skin color and, recently, hair curl.[18] What's needed is the development of simple validated tools. International consensus would allow universal adoption of objective assessments that could improve study quality and patient care. What now, as we march toward this objective ideal? We use ethnicity (eg, African ancestry, Afro-textured hair—only when clinically indicated) but we do so with the recognition that it is an imprecise surrogate that should be replaced as soon as possible.

Congratulations to South Africa, the Rainbow Nation, on 20 years of Democracy. May we each contribute to the greater good, daily...

Nonhlanhla P. Khumalo, MBChB, FCDerm, PhD
Head of Dermatology
Ward G23 Groote Schuur Hospital
Observatory 7925 and The University of Cape Town
Cape Town, Western Province
South Africa

E-mail address:
n.khumalo@uct.ac.za

REFERENCES

1. Everett BG, Rehkopf DH, Rogers RG. The nonlinear relationship between education and mortality: an examination of cohort, race/ethnic, and gender differences. Popul Res Policy Rev 2013;32(6).
2. Ringold S, Beukelman T, Nigrovic PA, et al. Race, ethnicity, and disease outcomes in juvenile idiopathic arthritis: a cross-sectional analysis of the Childhood Arthritis and Rheumatology Research Alliance (CARRA) Registry. J Rheumatol 2013; 40(6):936–42.
3. Bleil ME, Gregorich SE, Adler NE, et al. Race/ethnic disparities in reproductive age: an examination of ovarian reserve estimates across four race/ethnic groups of healthy, regularly cycling women. Fertil Steril 2014;101(1):199–207.
4. Morris AA, Cole RT, Veledar E, et al. Influence of race/ethnic differences in pre-transplantation panel reactive antibody on outcomes in heart transplant recipients. J Am Coll Cardiol 2013;62(24):2308–15.
5. Gayman MD, Cislo AM, Goidel AR, et al. SES and race-ethnic differences in the stress-buffering effects of coping resources among young adults. Ethn Health 2013.

6. Shin MH, Zmuda JM, Barrett-Connor E, et al. Race/ethnic differences in associations between bone mineral density and fracture history in older men. Osteoporos Int 2013.

7. Spanakis EK, Golden SH. Race/ethnic difference in diabetes and diabetic complications. Curr Diab Rep 2013;13(6):814–23.

8. Powell R, Davidson D, Divers J, et al. Genetic ancestry and the relationship of cigarette smoking to lung function and percent emphysema in four race/ethnic groups: a cross-sectional study. Thorax 2013;68(7):634–42.

9. Marquez-Magana L, Samayoa C, Umanzor C. Debunking 'race' and asserting social determinants as primary causes of cancer health disparities: outcomes of a science education activity for teens. J Cancer Educ 2013;28(2):314–8.

10. Williams DR, Earl TR. Commentary: race and mental health—more questions than answers. Int J Epidemiol 2007;36(4):758–60.

11. Hoover EL. There is no scientific rationale for race-based research. J Natl Med Assoc 2007;99(6):690–2.

12. Williams HC. Have you ever seen an Asian/Pacific Islander? Arch Dermatol 2002;138(5):673–4.

13. Golwala HB, Thadani U, Liang L, et al. Use of hydralazine-isosorbide dinitrate combination in African American and other race/ethnic group patients with heart failure and reduced left ventricular ejection fraction. J Am Heart Assoc 2013;2(4):e000214.

14. Bigby M, Thaler D. Describing patients' "race" in clinical presentations should be abandoned. J Am Acad Dermatol 2006;54(6):1074–6.

15. Bloche MG. Health care disparities—science, politics, and race. N Engl J Med 2004;350(15):1568–70.

16. Chaplin G, Jablonski NG. Hemispheric difference in human skin color. Am J Phys Anthropol 1998;107(2):221–3 [discussion: 223–4].

17. Jablonski NG, Chaplin G. The evolution of human skin coloration. J Hum Evol 2000;39(1):57–106.

18. Loussouarn G, Garcel AL, Lozano I, et al. Worldwide diversity of hair curliness: a new method of assessment. Int J Dermatol 2007;46(Suppl 1):2–6.

19. Parsa A, Kao WH, Xie D, et al. APOL1 risk variants, race, and progression of chronic kidney disease. N Engl J Med 2013;369(23):2183–96.

The Evolution of Skin Pigmentation and Hair Texture in People of African Ancestry

Nina G. Jablonski, PhD[a],*, George Chaplin, MSc[a,b]

KEYWORDS

• Melanin • Eumelanin • Ultraviolet radiation • *MC1R* • Afro-textured hair • Thermoregulation
• African American

KEY POINTS

- Variability in skin pigmentation phenotypes in African and African-admixed populations has not been well documented or genetically characterized.
- Afro-textured hair is a shared characteristic of most African and African-admixed people, and may represent an adaptation to protect the brain against thermal stress.
- Vitamin D deficiency is a risk for darkly pigmented people because of the natural sunscreening properties of eumelanin and the increased prevalence of indoor living.
- Use of race categories is ill-advised because of the genetic heterogeneity and socially constructed nature of races.

Our species, *Homo sapiens*, evolved in Africa, and humanity's highest levels of genetic diversity are maintained there today.[1] Underlying genetic diversity combined with the great range of solar regimes and climatic conditions found in Africa has contributed to a wide range of human integumentary phenotypes within the continent. Millions of Africans have moved, both voluntarily and involuntarily, to other continents in the past 2000 years, and the range of integumentary phenotypes among admixed African diaspora populations is enormous. In this contribution, we do not catalog this variation, but provide basic evolutionary background as to how it developed in the first place.

DIVERSITY OF INTEGUMENTARY PHENOTYPES WITHIN AFRICA

Africa has been a crucible of human diversification because of the length of human habitation there, and because of the continent's great size, environmental history, and past and present ecological diversity. Africa is the only continent that spans nearly 70° of latitude, thus containing an enormous range of solar radiation regimes. The continent's modern environmental mosaic first emerged about 20,000 years before present (BP) with the onset of more arid conditions across the continent. Formation and expansion of sand dunes along the southern margin of the Sahara and dramatic reductions in areas occupied by tropical forests proceeded until about 12,000 years BP.[2] Phases of increased wetness ("lacustrine phases") followed, from about 10,000 to 4000 years BP, during which the Sahara shrank and tropical forests rebounded.[2] Africa today exhibits a long and high elevational rise to the east along the Rift Valley that modifies the predominant global westerly humid air flow and creates a short seasonal monsoon. The specific effects of these environmental changes on

Disclosure: N.G. Jablonski is a member of the Scientific Advisory Board of L'Oreal.
[a] Department of Anthropology, The Pennsylvania State University, 409 Carpenter Building, University Park, PA 16802, USA; [b] Department of Geography, The Pennsylvania State University, 409 Carpenter Building, University Park, PA 16802, USA
* Corresponding author.
E-mail address: ngj2@psu.edu

derm.theclinics.com

human populations in Africa are not understood fully, but there is little doubt that they created opportunities for human biologic and cultural diversification by erecting and then eliminating geographic barriers to north-south and east-west migration. These changes alternately increased opportunities for the action of genetic drift and gene flow, such as across the Sahel corridor,[1] and created conditions under which biologic and cultural adaptations to rapid environmental change were promoted. Together, these factors contributed to the evolution of a large African population with a highly subdivided genetic structure.[3] The migration event that contributed most significantly to the establishment of the modern genetic landscape of Africa, including gene flow between once-isolated populations, was the expansion across Africa of the Bantu-language–speaking agriculturalists from near the Nigerian/Cameroonian highlands beginning approximately 3000 years BP.[1,3] This series of movements has resulted in overprinting of the original latitudinal cline of skin pigmentation, specifically, in the movement into southern Africa of equatorial peoples who are more darkly pigmented than the original moderately pigmented inhabitants.

Skin pigmentation is visibly different and measurably variable across Africa (**Fig. 1**). Diversity of environmental conditions, especially of ultraviolet radiation (UVR) regimes, along with population histories (including migrations) are the ultimate evolutionary causes of this diversity, but the specific and proximate genomic causes have not been elucidated fully. Studies of the genetics of skin pigmentation have focused on the significance of the virtual lack of variation in the sequence of the melanocortin 1 receptor (*MC1R*) locus in Africa,[4–7] compared with the extensive variation among African populations found elsewhere in the genome.[8] Between populations and individuals of African or African-admixed ancestry, differences in skin tone and the relative darkness of skin are due primarily to differences in the ratio of eumelanin to pheomelanin in the skin[9,10] that are regulated in part by the 8818G allele of the agouti signaling protein (*ASIP*) gene.[11] Subtle differences in skin tone are due to complex mixtures of melanin polymers and to the size and reflectance properties of the melanosomes in which the pigments are packaged.[12] Phenotypic differences in skin tone among and between people of African ancestry are incompletely known (see **Fig. 1**) and their genetic basis is inadequately understood.

Skin conditions affecting pigmentation produce highly visible disease states in normally darkly pigmented people. Of these, oculocutaneous albinism of the tyrosine-positive type (*OCA2*) is the most common that afflicts Africans and that has a genetic component. *OCA2* has been reported to occur at a prevalence approaching 1 in 1000 in some groups in Zimbabwe and South Africa, because of consanguinity and founder effects.[13,14] Individuals affected by albinism experience all the harmful effects of UVR exposure, including skin cancer, and face significant social ostracism, even death, because of their condition.[13–16] It has recently been suggested that the deleterious *OCA2* allele may be maintained in African populations as a balancing polymorphism, with the common deletion allele possibly conferring resistance to susceptibility to leprosy.[17]

Little is known about the evolution and diversification of human scalp hair phenotypes,[18] including the diversity that exists within Africa. Differences in hair color within Africa are minor and may represent pleiotropic effects of skin pigmentation genes.[12,19] Slight differences in hair form, growth characteristics, and susceptibility to breakage exist but have not been documented systematically. Sub-Saharan Africans generally exhibit tightly curled or Afro-textured hair and northern populations exhibit less tightly or loosely curled hair, but in all African populations, the hair shaft is elliptical in cross-section. The curliness of the hair shaft is caused by retrocurvature of the hair bulb, which gives rise to an asymmetrical S-shape of the hair follicle.[18] The continent-wide distribution of Afro-textured hair indicates that this is the ancestral condition for modern humans. Hrdy, who was one of the first to systematically characterize the morphology of human hair, speculated that hair form was determined by multiple genes, and that the tightly curly hair form had evolved convergently in African and Melanesian populations.[20,21] Progress has been made since then in the morphologic characterization of hair form,[22] but the genetic basis of hair form is still largely unknown. Symmetric hair follicles and generally straighter scalp hair shafts characterize Eurasian populations; the straight and thick hair shafts common to most East Asians are caused by a variant of the ectodysplasin receptor, *EDARV370A*.[23]

THE INFLUENCE OF NATURAL SELECTION ON INTEGUMENTARY PHENOTYPES

Throughout most of the history of the genus *Homo*, roughly 2 million years, naked skin has been the primary interface between our bodies and the environment.[24] The major speciation events leading to the emergence of *Homo sapiens* occurred at or near the equator in Africa, where levels of UVR are high throughout the year. Within

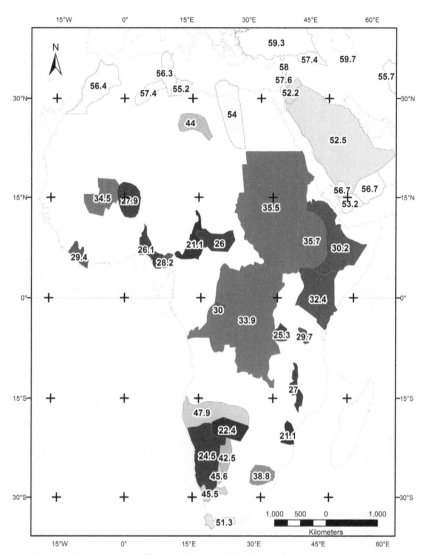

Fig. 1. Variation in human skin tones in Africa, as illustrated by skin reflectance values. The numbers within each polygon are the values for the reflectance of red light (685 nm) from the skin. (*Data from* Jablonski NG, Chaplin G. The evolution of human skin coloration. J Hum Evol 2000;39(1):57–106; and Chaplin G. Geographic distribution of environmental factors influencing human skin coloration. Am J Phys Anthropol 2004;125(3):292–302.)

the tropics, UVR levels potentially can be lowered by clouds and humidity, but otherwise the equinoctial peaks of UVB (medium wavelength UVR) caused by the earth's orbit around the sun are the most biologically significant sources of variation.[25] The intensity of UVB in sunlight is not perfectly correlated with heat produced by sunlight. Africa's UVB regimes vary according to latitude, but also are affected greatly by humidity and cloud cover (**Fig. 2**). High levels of atmospheric moisture contribute to generally lower levels of UVR, especially UVB, over western and central equatorial Africa, whereas negligible levels of atmospheric moisture contribute to extremely

high levels over the Sahara and the Namib, and much of eastern and northeastern Africa.

The many deleterious effects of UVR on biologic systems have promoted the evolution of complex processes of protection and repair, including protective pigmentation, DNA repair mechanisms, and means of neutralizing reactive oxygen species. Variation in UVR accounts for 86% of the observed variation in human skin pigmentation as measured by skin reflectance.[26,27] The stable clinal arrangement of human skin pigmentation that existed before the modern era of human migrations indicates the action of stabilizing selection over a spatially varying optimum condition.[28]

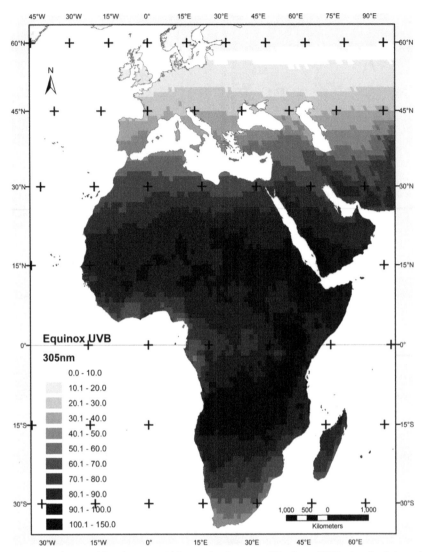

Fig. 2. Variation in UVB (305 nm) levels across Africa at the Autumnal Equinox (22 September), based on remotely sensed data collected by the NASA TOMS 7 satellite. Details of methodology are discussed elsewhere.[26]

The evolution of darkly pigmented, eumelanin-rich, naked skin, which is capable of tanning on exposure to UVR, was one of the key innovations of human biologic evolution. Constitutive dark pigmentation and capabilities for development of facultative dark pigmentation through tanning evolved independently in multiple human lineages[11,29] in response to high UVR regimes. Many reasons for the evolution of protective dark pigmentation have been proposed (as reviewed elsewhere[30]), but conservation of folate is supported by the largest body of evidence. The unique and critical roles played by folate and its metabolically active form, 5-methyltetrahydrofolate (5-MTHF), in DNA biosynthesis, repair, and methylation[25,26,31] and in the inhibition and repair of photosensitization-induced DNA strand breaks[32] imply that mechanisms to conserve folate and 5-MTHF in the presence of UVR would have been promoted by natural selection. Exposure of unprotected skin to UVR creates high demand for folate and 5-MTHF, which is further heightened during periods of rapid cell division, such as embryogenesis and spermatogenesis.[25] Exposure of the skin to UVR leads to direct photolysis of 5-MTHF in the presence of the endogenous photosensitizers riboflavin and uroporphyrin.[33,34] Serum folate levels undergo statistically significant decline in people following exposure to clinical doses of narrow-band UVB administered over the course of 3 weeks,[35] but not consistently after the same pattern of exposure to UVA.[36] Wavelength-specific photolysis appears to affect circulating levels of folate and

5-MTHF, but these levels are also certainly influenced by many other factors, including the polymorphic genes regulating folate and 5-MTHF metabolism, epigenetic modification of such genes, dietary folate consumption, and other factors, such as ethanol consumption.[37–39]

Human skin color is the product of 2 clines produced by natural selection to adjust levels of constitutive pigmentation to levels of UVR. Protective, eumelanin-rich skin pigmentation was the original condition for the genus Homo and has been maintained by stabilizing selection on combinations of different genes as an adaptation to high levels of UVR. Dark pigmentation is not disadvantageous from a thermoregulatory perspective to individuals living and exercising in sunny or arid environments. The heat-absorbing properties of eumelanin lead to darkly pigmented individuals showing higher core temperatures than lightly pigmented individuals after prolonged vigorous exercise, but no difference in evaporated sweat or in heat storage, which is balanced by increased long-wave radiation to the environment.[40,41] The genetic basis for skin pigmentation has been reviewed recently elsewhere.[42–44]

The continuously varying cline of eumelanin pigment in human skin from the equator to the poles is best explained as an adaptation for the maintenance of adequate levels of vitamin D in the body under conditions of seasonal or low UVR.[26,45,46] Vitamin D_3 is made in the skin when UVB (290–310 nm) penetrates the skin and is absorbed by 7-dehydrocholesterol (7-DHC) in the epidermis and dermis to form previtamin D_3. The potential for photosynthesis of vitamin D_3 in the skin depends on many environmental and personal factors: solar zenith angle (which varies according to season, latitude, and time of day), local humidity and pollution levels and weather conditions, the amount and distribution of eumelanin in the skin, and the thickness of the stratum corneum.[47–49] The importance of vitamin D_3 production as a selective force in the evolution of skin pigmentation has been reviewed elsewhere.[26,50,51] Because the vitamin D endocrine system is involved in the regulation of many independent biologic processes, including bone metabolism, the innate immune response, cell proliferation, and differentiation,[52–54] positive selection for maintenance of vitamin D production capability under highly seasonal or low average UVB levels has been a major determinant of human skin pigmentation phenotypes.[50,55] Most of the body's vitamin D is produced in the skin and does not come from dietary sources.[56] Dark pigmentation can be a risk factor for vitamin D deficiency when individuals do not receive sufficient UVR exposure to produce adequate levels of vitamin D. This can be the result of migration, indoor living, lack of outdoor activity, routine wearing of concealing clothing, or combinations of these factors that often exist in urban environments.[26,51] The clinical presentation of vitamin D deficiency depends not only on sun exposure and diet, but on genetic factors that affect the production, metabolism, and storage of vitamin D. The vitamin D endocrine system is regulated by many genes, including the vitamin D receptor locus (VDR), the vitamin D binding protein locus (VDBP), and those controlling the production of enzymes required for vitamin D synthesis and metabolism, such as CYP27B1 and CYP24A1.[57] Polymorphisms in these genes can have important consequences, but the functional significance of this variability is still not adequately known.[58] Vitamin D deficiency manifests itself in different ways depending on its duration, severity, and the interval in the life course when it strikes. Among the most serious potential consequences of vitamin D deficiency established for African, African diaspora, or African-admixed populations are elevated risks of nutritional rickets in children,[59] and of aggressive breast cancer[60] and tuberculosis in adults.[61,62] Vitamin D deficiency also aggravates problems of obesity and insulin resistance in the same populations[63,64]; patterns of comorbidity between vitamin D deficiency and type 2 diabetes mellitus and tuberculosis are not well understood.

In contrast to the situation for skin pigmentation, considerably less has been researched or written on the evolution of hair color and hair form. Most studies to date have dealt with the proximate genetic mechanisms responsible for producing lightly colored hair variants, and have focused especially on characterization of polymorphic MC1R loci and their associated phenotypes.[12,65] The operation of natural and/or sexual selection on hair color phenotypes has been proposed,[66] but not rigorously tested. Even less has been documented on the functional and evolutionary significance of hair form. Although hair form is almost certainly related to thermoregulation and the importance of keeping the head cool during exercise and under hot environmental conditions,[24,30] comparative studies of the effects of different hair forms on scalp and body temperature have not been conducted. Studies of the properties of bird plumage and mammal coats indicate that the color and the microstructure and microoptical properties of feathers or hairs, as well as the degree to which these appendages can be elevated by piloerection or passive lofting, contribute to the radiative heat loads that homeotherms acquire from solar radiation.[67,68] Humans evolved functional hairlessness on most of their bodies probably as the result of selection for enhanced eccrine sweating and the cooling benefits associated with the evaporation of sweat.[24,30] The presence of scalp hair in contrast to no scalp hair reduces environmental heat stress and reduces the total body sweat rate.[69] In the only experimental study of its kind, hair length and style were found to affect sweat rate and total body mass when humans were exposed to high environmental temperatures in a climate chamber.[70] Individuals with short straight hair and shorter permed hair had lower sweat rates and experienced less loss of total body mass after heat exposure.[70] Together with the evidence from studies of heat gain and loss in birds and nonhuman mammals, these findings suggest that short, curly, Afro-textured hair evolved because it can maintain a boundary layer of cooler, dryer air near the scalp, and thereby protect the thermogenic and thermosensitive brain. This hypothesis warrants experimental testing.

INTEGUMENTARY PHENOTYPES AND RACE

Skin color has been the primary feature used to classify people into groups or races. The first scientific classification of humans, written by Carolus Linneaus and published in 1738, placed people into 4 unranked "types" based on skin color and continent of origin. By 1758, Linneaus' classification further defined people by eye color and hair texture, and by general traits of character and disposition that accorded with the prevailing climatic theory of human diversity.[16] These ideas were embraced and extended by the philosopher Immanuel Kant, who was the first to define human "races" as fixed natural entities in his essay of 1775, "On the different human races."[16] Kant's classification differed from that of Linneaus in being explicitly hierarchical and based on skin color, which Kant viewed as a trait that denoted personality and morality. Kant equated skin color with character, and propagated ideas that lighter-colored races were superior and darker-colored ones inferior.[16] Because of his immense reputation, Kant was instrumental in establishing the "color meme," which profoundly affected attitudes toward the nature and meaning of human physical differences.[71] The persistence of racism and colorism has contributed to the promotion of skin lightening and the widespread use and abuse of skin bleaching agents among African and African-admixed populations worldwide.[16,72,73]

The nonexistence of human races is a scientific fact, which is based on the observations that similar "racial characteristics," such as skin color, have evolved multiple times, that such characteristics are generally not genetically linked to one another, and that patterns of phenotypic and genotypic diversity are not exclusive but extensively overlapping. Genomic research has revealed geographic clustering of some traits, but social factors alone have constructed and maintained races at different times and in different places.[16,74–76] There is an urgent need for clinical researchers and practicing physicians to recognize that the continued use of racial categories in medicine is inaccurate and irresponsible because it reinforces the existence of socially constructed categories, and fails to recognize the highly genetically heterogeneous nature of most human populations, including African and African-admixed groups. Most human populations today are heterogeneous and genetically admixed, and self-identified ancestry often does not reflect genetic ancestry accurately.[77,78] Many of the world's largest cities today on all inhabited continents have large proportions of people with African ancestry, and the genetic heterogeneity of this group must not be underestimated.

SUMMARY

Africa is home to the highest levels of human genetic diversity because of our species' long evolutionary history there, and because of the continent's large size, environmental diversity, and complex histories of human migration and isolation. The diversity of human skin pigmentation and hair texture phenotypes within Africa has not been well documented. Skin pigmentation within Africa generally varies by latitude, but the pattern has been overprinted by the migration of equatorial Bantu-language–speaking agriculturalists into eastern and southern Africa in the past 5000 years. The genetic basis of different skin tones among people of African ancestry has not been elucidated thoroughly. Dark pigmentation confers excellent protection against high levels of UVR, but predisposes individuals to vitamin D deficiency, especially those with indoor lifestyles. Afro-textured hair characterizes all African populations and is the likely ancestral condition for humans. It may have evolved as thermoregulatory adaptation to help keep the scalp and brain cool under conditions of high environmental heat and strenuous exercise. The evolution of integumentary phenotypes is characterized by widespread parallelism. For this and other reasons, skin color and hair texture cannot be used to classify people into races. The use of race to classify human groups in clinical contexts is ill-advised because of the highly genetically heterogeneous nature of most human populations, including African and African-admixed groups, and because races are socially constructed categories specific to particular times and places.

ACKNOWLEDGMENTS

We are grateful to Nonhlanhla Khumalo for inviting us to contribute to this special issue of *Dermatologic Clinics*. We thank Tess Wilson for help in obtaining bibliographic materials, and for all logistical matters related to manuscript preparation and submission. Jablonski is grateful to Ophelia Dadzie for discussions on the evolution and functional significance of Afro-textured hair.

REFERENCES

1. Tishkoff SA, Reed FA, Friedlaender FR, et al. The genetic structure and history of Africans and African Americans. Science 2009;324(5930):1035–44.
2. Nicholson SE, Flohn H. Holocene. Clim Change 1980;2(4):313–48.
3. Tishkoff SA, Verrelli BC. Patterns of human genetic diversity: implications for human evolutionary history and disease. Annu Rev Genomics Hum Genet 2003;4:293–340.
4. Harding RM, Healy E, Ray AJ, et al. Evidence for variable selective pressures at MC1R. Am J Hum Genet 2000;66:1351–61.
5. Sturm RA, Duffy DL, Box NF, et al. Genetic association and cellular function of MC1R variant alleles in human pigmentation. Ann N Y Acad Sci 2003; 994:348–58.
6. Gerstenblith MR, Goldstein AM, Fargnoli MC, et al. Comprehensive evaluation of allele frequency differences of MC1R variants across populations. Hum Mutat 2007;28(5):495–505.
7. John PR, Makova K, Li WH, et al. DNA polymorphism and selection at the melanocortin-1 receptor gene in normally pigmented southern African individuals. Ann N Y Acad Sci 2003;994:299–306.
8. Sturm RA, Box NF, Ramsay M. Human pigmentation genetics: the difference is only skin deep. Bioessays 1998;20(9):712–21.
9. Barsh GS. What controls variation in human skin color? PLoS Biol 2003;1(1):e27.
10. Alaluf S, Atkins D, Barrett K, et al. Ethnic variation in melanin content and composition in photoexposed and photoprotected human skin. Pigment Cell Res 2002;15(2):112–8.
11. Bonilla C, Boxill LA, McDonald S, et al. The 8818G allele of the agouti signaling protein (ASIP) gene is ancestral and is associated with darker skin color in African Americans. Hum Genet 2005;116(5): 402–6.
12. Rees JL. Genetics of hair and skin color. Annu Rev Genet 2003;37:67–90.
13. Hong E, Zeeb H, Repacholi M. Albinism in Africa as a public health issue. BMC Public Health 2006; 6(1):212–8.
14. Cruz-Inigo AE, Ladizinski B, Sethi A. Albinism in Africa: stigma, slaughter and awareness campaigns. Dermatol Clin 2011;29(1):79–87.
15. Gettleman J. Albinos being "hunted" for their body parts. The Seattle Times; 2008. Nation & World.
16. Jablonski NG. Living color: the biological and social meaning of skin color. Berkeley (CA): University of California Press; 2012.
17. Tuli AM, Valenzuela RK, Kamugisha E, et al. Albinism and disease causing pathogens in Tanzania: are alleles that are associated with OCA2 being maintained by balancing selection? Med Hypotheses 2012;79(6):875–8.
18. Westgate GE, Botchkareva NV, Tobin DJ. The biology of hair diversity. Int J Cosmet Sci 2013; 35(4):329–36.
19. Han J, Kraft P, Nan H, et al. A genome-wide association study identifies novel alleles associated with hair color and skin pigmentation. PLoS Genet 2008; 4(5):e1000074.
20. Hrdy D. Quantitative hair form variation in seven populations. Am J Phys Anthropol 1973;39(1): 7–17.
21. Hrdy DB, Baden HP, Lee LD, et al. Frequency of an electrophoretic variant of hair alpha keratin in human populations. Am J Hum Genet 1977;29(1): 98–100.
22. De La Mettrie R, Saint-Léger D, Loussouarn G, et al. Shape variability and classification of human hair: a worldwide approach. Hum Biol 2007;79(3): 265–81.
23. Kamberov Yana G, Wang S, Tan J, et al. Modeling recent human evolution in mice by expression of a selected EDAR variant. Cell 2013;152(4):691–702.
24. Jablonski NG. Skin: a natural history. Berkeley (CA): University of California Press; 2006.
25. Jablonski NG, Chaplin G. Human skin pigmentation as an adaptation to UV radiation. Proc Natl Acad Sci U S A 2010;107(Suppl 2):8962–8.
26. Jablonski NG, Chaplin G. The evolution of human skin coloration. J Hum Evol 2000;39(1):57–106.
27. Chaplin G. Geographic distribution of environmental factors influencing human skin coloration. Am J Phys Anthropol 2004;125(3):292–302.
28. Jablonski NG. Skin coloration. In: Muehlenbein MI, editor. Human evolutionary biology. Cambridge (United Kingdom): Cambridge University Press; 2010. p. 192–213.
29. Quillen EE, Bauchet M, Bigham AW, et al. OPRM1 and EGFR contribute to skin pigmentation differences between Indigenous Americans and Europeans. Hum Genet 2012;131(7):1073–80.

30. Jablonski NG. The evolution of human skin and skin color. Annu Rev Anthropol 2004;33:585–623.

31. Branda RF, Eaton JW. Skin color and nutrient photolysis: an evolutionary hypothesis. Science 1978;201(4356):625–6.

32. Offer T, Ames BN, Bailey SW, et al. 5-Methyltetrahydrofolate inhibits photosensitization reactions and strand breaks in DNA. FASEB J 2007;21(9):2101–7.

33. Tam TT, Juzeniene A, Steindal AH, et al. Photodegradation of 5-methyltetrahydrofolate in the presence of uroporphyrin. J Photochem Photobiol B 2009;94(3):201–4.

34. Steindal AH, Tam TT, Lu XY, et al. 5-Methyltetrahydrofolate is photosensitive in the presence of riboflavin. Photochem Photobiol Sci 2008;7(7):814–8.

35. Shaheen MA, Abdel Fattah NS, El-Borhamy MI. Analysis of serum folate levels after narrow band UVB exposure. Egyptian Dermatology Online Journal 2006;2(1):15.

36. Gambichler T, Sauermann K, Bader A, et al. Serum folate levels after UVA exposure: a two-group parallel randomised controlled trial. BMC Dermatol 2001;1(1):8.

37. Borradale DC, Kimlin MG. Folate degradation due to ultraviolet radiation: possible implications for human health and nutrition. Nutr Rev 2012;70(7):414–22.

38. Lucock M, Glanville T, Ovadia L, et al. Photoperiod at conception predicts C677T-MTHFR genotype: a novel gene-environment interaction. Am J Human Biol 2010;22(4):484–9.

39. Lucock M, Glanville T, Yates Z, et al. Solar cycle predicts folate-sensitive neonatal genotypes at discrete phases of the first trimester of pregnancy: a novel folate-related human embryo loss hypothesis. Med Hypotheses 2012;79(2):210–5.

40. Baker PT. The biological adaptation of man to hot deserts. Am Nat 1958;92(867):337–57.

41. Baker PT. Racial differences in heat tolerance. Am J Phys Anthropol 1958;16(3):287–305.

42. Sturm RA. Molecular genetics of human pigmentation diversity. Hum Mol Genet 2009;18(R1):R9–17.

43. Rees JL, Harding RM. Understanding the evolution of human pigmentation: recent contributions from population genetics. J Invest Dermatol 2012;132(3):846–53.

44. Sturm RA, Duffy DL. Human pigmentation genes under environmental selection. Genome Biol 2012;13(9):1–15.

45. Murray FG. Pigmentation, sunlight, and nutritional disease. Am Anthropol 1934;36(3):438–45.

46. Loomis WF. Skin-pigment regulation of vitamin-D biosynthesis in man. Science 1967;157(3788):501–6.

47. Holick MF, MacLaughlin JA, Clark MB, et al. Photosynthesis of previtamin D3 in human skin and the physiologic consequences. Science 1980;210(4466):203–5.

48. Holick MF. Photosynthesis of vitamin D in the skin: effect of environmental and life-style variables. Fed Proc 1987;46(5):1876–82.

49. Lips P. Vitamin D physiology. Prog Biophys Mol Biol 2006;92(1):4–8.

50. Chaplin G, Jablonski NG. Vitamin D and the evolution of human depigmentation. Am J Phys Anthropol 2009;139(4):451–61.

51. Jablonski NG, Chaplin G. Human skin pigmentation, migration and disease susceptibility. Philos Trans R Soc Lond B Biol Sci 2012;367(1590):785–92.

52. Norman AW. From vitamin D to hormone D: fundamentals of the vitamin D endocrine system essential for good health. Am J Clin Nutr 2008;88(2):491S–9S.

53. Kostner K, Denzer N, Muller CS, et al. The relevance of vitamin D receptor (VDR) gene polymorphisms for cancer: a review of the literature. Anticancer Res 2009;29(9):3511–36.

54. Hossein-Nezhad A, Holick MF. Vitamin D for health: a global perspective. Mayo Clin Proc 2013;88(7):720–55.

55. Norton HL, Kittles RA, Parra E, et al. Genetic evidence for the convergent evolution of light skin in Europeans and East Asians. Mol Biol Evol 2007;24(3):710–22.

56. Chen TC, Chimeh F, Lu Z, et al. Factors that influence the cutaneous synthesis and dietary sources of vitamin D. Arch Biochem Biophys 2007;460(2):213–7.

57. Yao S, Zirpoli G, Bovbjerg DH, et al. Variants in the vitamin D pathway, serum levels of vitamin D, and estrogen receptor negative breast cancer among African-American women: a case-control study. Breast Cancer Res 2012;14(2):R58.

58. Uitterlinden AG, Fang Y, van Meurs JB, et al. Genetics and biology of vitamin D receptor polymorphisms. Gene 2004;338(2):143–56.

59. Pettifor JM. Nutritional rickets: pathogenesis and prevention. Pediatr Endocrinol Rev 2013;10(S2):347–53.

60. Yao S, Ambrosone CB. Associations between vitamin D deficiency and risk of aggressive breast cancer in African-American women. J Steroid Biochem Mol Biol 2013;136:337–41.

61. Martineau AR, Nhamoyebonde S, Oni T, et al. Reciprocal seasonal variation in vitamin D status and tuberculosis notifications in Cape Town, South Africa. Proc Natl Acad Sci U S A 2011;108(47):19013–7.

62. Coussens AK, Wilkinson RJ, Nikolayevskyy V, et al. Ethnic variation in inflammatory profile in tuberculosis. PLoS Pathog 2013;9(7):e1003468.

63. Renzaho AM, Nowson C, Kaur A, et al. Prevalence of vitamin D insufficiency and risk factors for type 2 diabetes and cardiovascular disease

among African migrant and refugee adults in Melbourne: a pilot study. Asia Pac J Clin Nutr 2011;20(3):397–403.

64. Harris SS, Pittas AG, Palermo NJ. A randomized, placebo-controlled trial of vitamin D supplementation to improve glycaemia in overweight and obese African Americans. Diabetes Obes Metab 2012; 14(9):789–94.

65. Sturm RA, Teasdale RD, Fox NF. Human pigmentation genes: identification, structure and consequences of polymorphic variation. Gene 2001; 277(1–2):49–62.

66. Frost P. European hair and eye color: a case of frequency-dependent sexual selection? Evol Hum Behav 2006;27(2):85–103.

67. Wolf BO, Walsberg GE. The role of the plumage in heat transfer processes of birds. Am Zool 2000; 40(4):575–84.

68. Walsberg GE. Consequences of skin color and fur properties for solar heat gain and ultraviolet irradiance in two mammals. J Comp Physiol B 1988; 158(2):213–21.

69. Coelho LG, Ferreira-Junior JB, Martini AR, et al. Head hair reduces sweat rate during exercise under the sun. Int J Sports Med 2010;31(11):779–83.

70. Kim MJ, Choi JW, Lee HK. Effect of hair style on human physiological responses in a hot environment. Paper presented at: Environmental Ergonomics: Proceedings of the 13th International Conference on Environmental Ergonomics. Boston, MA, August 2–7, 2009.

71. Jablonski NG. The struggle to overcome racism. New Sci 2012;(2880):26–9.

72. Hall R. The bleaching syndrome: African Americans' response to cultural domination vis-a-vis skin color. J Black Stud 1995;26(2):172–84.

73. Ladizinski B, Mistry N, Kundu RV. Widespread use of toxic skin lightening compounds: medical and psychosocial aspects. Dermatol Clin 2011;29(1): 111–23.

74. Long JC, Kittles RA. Human genetic diversity and the nonexistence of biological races. Hum Biol 2009;81(5–6):777–98.

75. Shiao JL, Bode T, Beyer A, et al. The genomic challenge to the social construction of race. Soc Theory 2012;30(2):67–88.

76. Soudien C. The modern seduction of race: Whither social constructionism? Transformation: Critical Perspectives on Southern Africa 2012;79:18–38.

77. Bonilla C, Gutierrez G, Parra EJ, et al. Admixture analysis of a rural population of the state of Guerrero, Mexico. Am J Phys Anthropol 2005;128(4): 861–9.

78. Klimentidis YC, Miller GF, Shriver MD. Genetic admixture, self-reported ethnicity, self-estimated admixture, and skin pigmentation among Hispanics and Native Americans. Am J Phys Anthropol 2009;138(4):375–83.

What's New in Objective Assessment and Treatment of Facial Hyperpigmentation?

Vanessa E. Molinar, BA[a],*, Susan C. Taylor, MD[b,c],
Amit G. Pandya, MD[d]

KEYWORDS

- Melasma • Postinflammatory hyperpigmentation • Dermatosis papulosa nigra
- Lichen planus pigmentosus • Erythema dyschromicum perstans
- Objective assessment of pigmentation • Treatment

KEY POINTS

- Facial hyperpigmentation is common and disfiguring in people of African ancestry.
- Melasma is the most studied with validated severity scoring tools; however, combination treatments are often required to improve efficacy.
- More work is required to develop and validate severity scoring tools and to elucidate effective treatments for postinflammatory hyperpigmentation and lichen planus pigmentosus.

INTRODUCTION

Hyperpigmentation, which commonly affects dark-skinned individuals, is often challenging to treat. Disorders of hyperpigmentation have been demonstrated to have a negative impact on quality of life.[1] Pigmentary disorders occur with greater frequency and severity in black populations and are a frequent reason for dermatologic consultation.[1–3] Halder and Nootheti[4] reported that pigmentary disorders (excluding vitiligo) were the third most common reason for dermatologic consultation among African American patients.[4] In a 2005 study by Alexis and colleagues,[5] pigmentary disorders ranked second in the 5 top diagnoses (acne, dyschromia, eczema, alopecia, and seborrheic dermatitis) in the black population.

Facial pigmentary disorders that are of greatest concern are melasma, postinflammatory hyper- or hypopigmentation, dermatosis papulosis nigra (DPN), seborrheic keratosis, lichen planus pigmentosus, and erythema dyschromicum perstans (EDP).[1,2]

OBJECTIVE ASSESSMENT—MELASMA

Clinical Findings

Melasma is characterized by irregular brown patches on sun-exposed skin, most commonly involving malar prominences, the forehead, the upper lip, the nose, and the chin (Fig. 1).[1,6] As discussed by Sheth and Pandya,[6] the centrofacial pattern is the most common pattern, characterized by lesions on the forehead, cheeks, nose, upper lip, or chin. The malar pattern consists of lesions primarily on cheeks and nose. The mandibular pattern consists of lesions on the ramus of the mandible.

Severity Scales

The Melasma Area and Severity Index (MASI) score is an outcome measure first developed and implemented by Kimbrough-Green and

[a] Paul L. Foster School of Medicine, Texas Tech University Health Sciences Center, 5001 El Paso Dr, El Paso, TX 79905, USA; [b] College of Physicians and Surgeons, Columbia University Medical Center, 630 W 168th Street, New York, NY 10032, USA; [c] Society Hill Dermatology, 932 Pine Street, Philadelphia, PA 19107, USA; [d] Department of Dermatology, University of Texas Southwestern Medical Center, 5939 Harry Hines Boulevard #300, Dallas, TX 75235, USA
* Corresponding author.
E-mail address: vanessa.molinar@ttuhsc.edu

Dermatol Clin 32 (2014) 123–135
http://dx.doi.org/10.1016/j.det.2013.12.008
0733-8635/14/$ – see front matter © 2014 Elsevier Inc. All rights reserved.

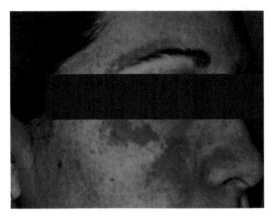

Fig. 1. Melasma of right cheek.

colleagues.[7] This index was based on a similar scoring system devised for psoriasis. The score is calculated by adding the sum of severity ratings for darkness and homogeneity, which is then multiplied by a value representing the area of involvement, for each of 4 facial areas, with a total score ranging from 0 to 48. The MASI is the most commonly used outcome measure for melasma trials, but, until recently, it had never been validated. A prospective study conducted by Pandya and colleagues[8] found that although the MASI demonstrated good reliability within and between raters, there were problems with 2 individual components of the MASI, namely the assessment of the chin and homogeneity of melasma lesions. Validation was performed by comparing the MASI with the melasma severity scale, mexameter scores, and area measurements. Homogeneity was the most difficult component to assess reliably. The researchers found that by removing the homogeneity parameter from the MASI, reliability and validity were not altered. Thus, the authors recommended removal of homogeneity from the MASI score altogether. Removal of the assessment of the chin was not recommended because it only represented 10% of the overall score, and variations in assessment of this area did not cause the MASI score to change significantly. This new assessment tool has been termed the modified MASI score and scores range from 0 to 24. Future studies are needed to assess the sensitivity of the modified MASI in objectively assessing change in melasma over time with treatment. The Taylor hyperpigmentation scale[9] was developed to assess hyperpigmentation in both a research and a clinical setting, requires minimal training, is easy to administer, and is inexpensive to perform. There are a possible of 100 different ratings using this scale, consisting of a series of laminated plastic cards that are printed in 10 different skin colors (S = J) and 10 gradations of pigment for each

skin type. In a pilot study using 24 subjects with Fitzpatrick skin types III–IV, the scale scored well for "ease of use" and "usefulness" for 8 of 10 evaluators. Six of 10 clinicians stated the scale had too few choices of skin color or hue, and 2 of 10 stated there were too many choices. Their feedback prompted the development of a modified scale that includes 15 skin hues or colors representing skin types I–IV.

Polarized light photography is useful in the assessment of dermal changes, including dermal melasma; however, it may be less useful in the assessment of epidermal pigmentation.[10] Accurate and reproducible readings of melasma can be obtained for the objective measurement of skin color with hand-held tristimulus reflectance colorimeters, such as the Photovolt Color Walk Colorimeter (Photovolt instruments, Minneapolis, MN, USA) and the Minolta Chromameter (Minolta, Osaka, Japan), as well as narrowband reflectance spectrophotometers such as DermaSpectrophotometer and the Mexameter. A previous study comparing the Minolta Chromameter, DermaSpectrophotometer (Cortex Technologies, Hadsund, Denmark), and the Mexameter demonstrated good day-to-day repeatability in melanin measurement (1% variability) for both the Chromameter and the Mexameter, but poor repeatability for the DermaSpectrometer (4% variability).[11] The authors found that all 3 instruments were able to characterize and quantify small changes in skin color. In addition, the investigators agreed with previous findings that the Chromameter was capable of measuring all colors, whereas reflectance spectrophotometers were effective at measuring intensity of erythema and melanin-induced pigmentation.[10,11] The use of reflectance spectroscopy in objectively determining the relationship between the L* value (Color Walk Colorimeter) and M index (DermaSpectrophotometer) has been previously investigated.[12] African American subjects with the darkest skin had the lowest L* values and the highest M indices, whereas the subjects of European ancestry with the lightest skin had high L* values and low M indices.

Finally, several techniques are now available for the objective assessment of pigmentation in melasma. Together with scoring methods to quantify subjective evaluations better, reliable outcome measures that can be used in melasma studies to produce reproducible results are now available.

PHARMACOLOGIC TREATMENT OPTIONS: MELASMA

Although multiple studies have focused on developing new therapies for treatment of melasma, there are few studies that focus treatment strategies specifically for patients with darker skin types. Sheth and Pandya[6,13] made recommendations based on US Preventive Service Task Force levels of evidence for grading clinical trials in managing melasma (Table 1).

In a vehicle-controlled clinical trial, investigators assessed the efficacy of 0.1% tretinoin cream in African American subjects with melasma applied daily for 10 months.[9] Objective measurement of skin color changes was measured with colorimetry (Chroma Meter-CR200 [Minolta, Osaka, Japan]), and histopathologic evaluation was also performed from a representative area of melasma pre- and posttreatment. MASI scores were calculated for each patient at baseline and at 24 and 40 weeks to assess melasma severity. Initial benefit was seen after 24 weeks of treatment, with 40% lightening toward normal skin color compared with 4% by the vehicle group. Tretinoin-induced reduction in epidermal pigment observed by histology did not significantly correlate with a reduction in either clinical or colorimetric lightening. The study did not find evidence of further hyperpigmentation in their patients.

Table 1
Current standard of treatment for managing melasma

	Primary Agent	Alternative Agent
First-line treatment	Triple combination products containing HQ, a retinoid, fluorinated steroid once daily, or HQ 4% twice daily for up to 6-mo periods	Azelaic acid
Adjuvant treatment	Ascorbic acid	Kojic acid
Second-line	Glycolic acid peels every 4–6 wk starting at 40% and increasing in concentration as tolerated	
Third-line	Fractional laser therapy	Intense pulsed light

Additional author recommendations include regular use of broad-spectrum photoprotection along with sun avoidance.

From Sheth VM, Pandya AG. Melasma: a comprehensive update: part II. J Am Acad Dermatol 2011;65(4):689–97; with permission.

This study demonstrates that although tretinoin is an effective treatment for melasma, it often produces irritation and requires a mean treatment duration of 6 months to demonstrate significant improvement; therefore, it is not considered a first-line therapy for melasma.

Other topical agents, such as adapalene, azelaic acid, kojic acid, ascorbic acid, arbutin/deoxyarbutin, licorice extract, and soy, have been investigated for either treatment of melasma or solar lentigines. However, clinical studies evaluating their efficacy in the treatment of melasma in skin phototypes IV–VI are necessary.[13] Similarly, the use of glycolic acid peels in clinical studies demonstrates variable efficacy and may cause various side effects that are undesirable, such as erythema, desquamation, and postinflammatory hyperpigmentation (PIH).[13–15] Adjunctive therapy with other chemical peels, such as 1% retinoic acid, Jessner solution, and salicylic acid, has not been shown to add long-term benefit in patients with melasma.

Combination Therapies

Topical therapies with a triple combination agent appear to be the most clinically efficacious treatment for patients with melasma.[13] A study on a combination formulation of 0.4% hydroquinone (HQ), 0.05% tretinoin, and 0.01% fluocinolone acetonide has not only shown significant success in achieving near-complete clearance compared with patients using dual-combination regimens, but also demonstrated significant improvement in MASI scores in 73% of black patients and 95% of black/Hispanic patients after 8 weeks of therapy.[16] Side effects were rated as mild; however, irritation can lead to development of PIH in patients with darker skin types. Thus, a decrease in the frequency of application is recommended in those who develop irritation.[13] In another small study, 50% of patients demonstrated subjective clinical improvement with a combination of 0.05% tretinoin, 0.05% triamcinolone acetonide, 6% HQ, and 0.1% ascorbic acid (Table 2).[17]

Surgical Treatments

Patients of darker skin types with melasma are at risk of PIH following laser treatment with Q-switched ruby, Erbium-yttrium-aluminum-garnet, and Q-switched alexandrite 755-nm lasers; therefore, these lasers are not generally recommended because of ineffectiveness and increased risk of adverse events.[1,13] Fractional laser therapy is the only laser treatment for melasma approved by the US Food and Drug Administration because it has shown promising results in a study evaluating

Table 2
Treatment, outcomes, and recommendations for managing melasma based on recommendations from Sheth and Pandya

Therapy	Treatment	Outcome	Comments
Monotherapy			
20% azelaic acid[22]	Twice daily for 24 wk	68.9% of participants (300) reported good or excellent results vs 43.7% in HQ group. Results statistically significant	36.5% in azelaic acid group reported adverse effects vs 12.7% in HQ group
5% ascorbic acid cream[23]	5% ascorbic acid cream on one side of face and 4% HQ cream on the other side daily for 16 wk	HQ demonstrated better response with subjective improvement of 93% good and excellent results vs 62% on ascorbic acid side, statistically significant result; however, colorimetry did not reach significance	Adverse effects reported in 68.7% with HQ vs 6.2% with ascorbic acid
Combination treatments			
4% HQ, 0.05% tretinoin, 0.01% fluocinolone acetonide[16]	Daily for 8 wk	26% of subjects treated with triple combination therapy achieved complete clearance vs 4.6 in other groups. Improvement subjectively assessed by investigators	Erythema, desquamation, burning, dryness, pruritus, and PIH in darker-skin types
0.05% tretinoin, 0.05% triamcinolone acetonide, 6% HQ, and 0.1% ascorbic acid[17]	Nightly for 8 wk. Evaluated at baseline and monthly during treatment	Moderate-to-significant improvement in 5 of 6 patients	Mild adverse events reported, including slight irritation reversible on discontinuation of treatment
2% kojic acid in gel + 10% glycolic acid + 2% HQ[24]	40 subjects treated with 2% KJ + 10% glycolic acid + 2% HQ to one-half of face, other half treated with same application minus KJ. Twice daily for 12 wk with SPF 15 sunscreen used daily	60% subjects improved in KJ group vs 47.5% in control, assessment subjective by investigators	Reported side effects include redness, stinging, and exfoliation
Chemical peels			
Glycolic acid[15]	Nightly serial peels in combination with topical azelaic acid 20% cream (bid) and 0.1% adapalene gel (qid) for 20 wk vs control group (topical azelaic acid + adapalene)	Statistically significant reduction in MASI scores compared with baseline in treatment group	Adverse events reported include mild-degree PIH, with clearance at the end of treatment

Abbreviation: KJ, kojic acid.

Adapted from Sheth VM, Pandya AG. Melasma: a comprehensive update: part II. J Am Acad Dermatol 2011;65(4):689–97; with permission.

its efficacy in 10 female subjects with skin types III–IV.[13,18] In this study, the 6 subjects with skin type III demonstrated good improvement to therapy, whereas the 4 subjects with skin type IV demonstrated fair improvement, without a correlation between histologic improvement and investigator-rated improvement. PIH was not observed in patients at a 3-month follow-up visit.

Nonablative fractional photothermolysis (NFP) is thought to eliminate both epidermal and dermal melanin by compromising the dermal-epidermal junction and disrupting dermal macrophages containing melanin. A recent prospective controlled single-blinded study investigating the efficacy of NFP for the treatment of melasma did not show increased benefit in treating melasma when compared with the lone application of broad-spectrum sunscreen.[19] Thus, the authors did not recommend the use of NFP in treating melasma and encouraged physicians to approach this method conservatively. Further studies with a larger sample size in darker skinned individuals are recommended for this method of treatment.

Intense pulse light (IPL) is a non-laser light source that has been studied alone and in combination with HQ for the treatment of melasma. Alone, authors have found a decrease in MASI scores from 15.2 to 5.2 after 4 sessions, and a further decrease to 4.5 at the 3-month follow-up.[20] Common side effects included temporary erythema and edema, and PIH. In a comparative study investigating the efficacy of IPL to 4% HQ, investigators found a 39.8% decrease in the relative melanin index after a total of 16 weeks of treatment, compared with an 11.6% decrease in those treated with topical therapy alone.[21] Although these studies have not included dark-skinned individuals, and caution should be used in these individuals, IPL has been recommended as an alternative third-line treatment for patients with melasma refractory to topical therapy alone (**Table 3**).[13]

Summary

Topical depigmenting agents, especially those that contain HQ in combination with a steroid and retinoid, are the most effective and safe for the treatment of melasma. Thus, first-line therapy for melasma should include triple combination products containing HQ, a retinoid, fluorinated steroid once daily, or HQ 4%, as recommended by Sheth and Pandya.[13] Studies investigating the efficacy of chemical peels, laser, and light therapies have produced mixed results and increase the risk of hyperpigmentation in darker-skinned individuals.

OBJECTIVE ASSESSMENT-PIH

PIH typically manifests as macules or patches at the site of previous inflammation, and the presence of a consistent history simplifies the

Table 3			
Treatment, outcomes, and recommendations for laser therapy for melasma			
Laser	Treatment Duration	Outcomes	Comments
NFP[19]	Pulse energy of 15 mJ/ microthermal zone (MTZ), total density 1048 MTZ/ cm², density per pass 131 MTZs/cm², 8 passes, and total coverage of 20%	In 51 patients, no significant reduction in PGA assessment compared with controls. Decrease MASI score in control group 1.4 ± 0.9 vs 0.6 ± 0.6 in treatment	No adverse events reported Investigators limited outcome measure in MASI as the primary outcome variable instead of spectroscopic analysis of hyperpigmentation before and after treatment
Intense pulsed light[20,21]	4 IPL sessions at 3-wk intervals, 3-mo follow-up visit assessment with MASI	77.5% of patients (69/89) demonstrated 51%–100% improvement by dermatologic evaluation. Mean MASI reduction from 15.2 to 4.5 at the 3-mo follow-up visit	Sunscreen before and after treatment. Minimal adverse events included transient edema and erythema
	IPL vs 4% HQ with sunscreen (control); 4 sessions at 4-wk intervals[21]	Relative melanin index demonstrated 39.8% improvement in IPL group vs 11.6% in control group	PIH reported in 2 patients and repigmentation

Adapted from Sheth VM, Pandya AG. Melasma: a comprehensive update: part II. J Am Acad Dermatol 2011;65(4):689–97; with permission.

diagnosis.[1,6] Acne vulgaris is a common cause of PIH (**Fig. 2**). The distribution of pigmentation can be epidermal, dermal, or mixed type.[1] Unlike dermal and mixed lesions, epidermal lesions tend to be well circumscribed and are enhanced under Wood lamp examination.

The postacne hyperpigmentation index, an outcome measure developed to provide a more accurate quantification of the severity of PIH in patients with PIH from acne, has been found to be reliable and validated against other measures.[25] This index measures darkness, size, and number of lesions, resulting in a score from 6 to 22. Histologic quantification of melanocytes is variable and has not been validated for PIH.[11] Noninvasive methodologies to quantify hyperpigmentation include high-resolution digital imaging systems and ultraviolet fluorescence photography. However, these techniques are limited in their ability to assess differences between pigmentation and inflammation and have not been validated. Imaging techniques do provide a reference value that may guide clinicians in determining therapeutic doses or to monitor response.

Although outcome measures for PIH in the past have not been validated or studied for reliability, new research is providing tools for investigators to obtain reproducible results. Standardized outcome measures that are then used for treatment studies would be a welcome addition to the dermatologist's armamentarium. Further investigations are recommended to develop methods for objective assessment in both research and clinical settings for the assessment of PIH.

PHARMACOLOGIC TREATMENT OPTIONS (PIH)

Initial management of PIH should address the underlying inflammatory dermatosis. However, the treatment initiated may have the potential to exacerbate the PIH by causing irritation.[3] Currently, the mainstay of treatment of PIH is HQ, either as monotherapy in concentrations from 2% to 4% or formulated combining retinoids, antioxidants, glycolic acid, steroids, or as sunscreen to increase efficacy. None of these treatment reports have used a validated outcome measure to determine improvement. Topical mequinol 2%-tretinoin 0.01% has been shown to be just as efficacious as 4% HQ in a comparative study with 61 skin-of-color patients with mild-to-moderate facial PIH.[26] The use of 0.1% tretinoin in black patients with PIH has also been shown to lighten lesions of PIH; however, 50% of patients developed retinoid dermatitis.[27] Once-daily application of 0.1% tazarotene cream has demonstrated effectiveness in the treatment of PIH as well as the treatment of acne in darker skinned individuals.[28] Adapalene (0.1%–0.3%) formulated in cream or gel also appears to be effective and safe in the treatment of acne-induced PIH.[3] Other lightening agents, such as azelaic acid, kojic acid, arbutin, niacinamide, N-acetylglucosamine, ascorbic acid, licorice, and soy, require further, larger controlled studies examining their efficacy in the treatment of PIH in this patient population and all treatments should be repeated using validated outcome measures.[3,29]

Chemical peels have been generally well tolerated with good results in the treatment of PIH; however, one must be careful in selecting the proper chemical peel to avoid irritation and worsening of PIH.[30] Glycolic acid, which induces epidermolysis, has been investigated in African Americans for facial PIH, but failed to demonstrate a significant difference compared with controls.[31] Other superficial chemical peels, such as trichloracetic acid or Jessner's solution, lack clinical evidence supporting their use for PIH in skin of color.[3]

Nonpharmacologic Treatment Options

Photoprotection is an integral component in the treatment of PIH and is aimed at preventing the disorder from worsening.[3] Sun avoidance and use of broad-spectrum sunscreens are essential, especially in individuals with higher skin phototypes who may not be aware of the darkening effects UV radiation has on hyperpigmentation.[1,3] Adjunctive treatment with a daily dose of 1000 IU vitamin D is recommended in this population because they are at increased risk of vitamin D deficiency.[3,32] Cosmetic camouflage is also useful in concealing hyperpigmentation, alleviating patient's distress regarding their appearance and quality of life; this is particularly useful in darker

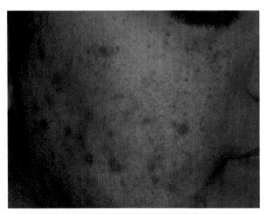

Fig. 2. Postinflammatory hyperpigmentation from acne vulgaris.

skinned individuals where pigmentary changes are more noticeable.

Combination Therapies

Tranexamic acid (TXA) is a lysine analogue that has been shown to have antiplasmin activity, which prevents UV-induced pigmentation.[29] Niacinamide is a member of the vitamin B_3 family, which has shown promising results in the inhibition of melanosome transfer from melanocytes to keratinocytes. In an 8-week, prospective, randomized, double-blind, vehicle controlled study, investigators studied the efficacy of formulated combination of topical 2% TXA and 2% niacinamide in the treatment of facial hyperpigmentation. Hyperpigmentation was assessed with a mexameter at baseline, week 4, and week 8 of the study. Photographs were graded according to a pigment intensity score (1–10 scale), and skin lightness was assessed with a chromameter. Melanin index scores decreased significantly from baseline at both 4 and 8 weeks ($P<.001$ and $P<.001$, respectively). Skin lightening effects assessed by chromameter also demonstrated statistical significance, with increased lightening compared with control group of 2.02% versus 0.25% at week 8 ($P = .018$). No serious adverse effects were reported by the patients in this study. Although this clinical study did not evaluate the use of TXA and niacinamide specifically in PIH in higher skin phototypes, their results suggest a promising therapy in the treatment of facial hyperpigmentation with minimal adverse effects.

The use of oral TXA for the prophylaxis of laser-induced PIH has also been investigated in a single-center, randomized, parallel-group study.[33] Thirty-two participants with solar lentigines with or without melasma were treated with either 750 mg/d of TXA for 4 weeks after Q-switched Ruby laser treatment or laser treatment without TXA. Objective assessment included use of spectrophotometry (Mexameter MX 16) at baseline, and at 2 and 4 weeks after treatment. The study did not demonstrate statistically significant differences between the TXA+ and TXA− group regarding the degree of PIH after laser treatment. The authors suggested insufficient dose and time to achieve significant prophylaxis of PIH after laser treatment. This method of treatment has not been assessed in larger populations, including darker skinned individuals.

A combination formulation of topical gel clindamycin 1.2% and tretinoin 0.025% has also been recently investigated in a 12-week, double-blind, randomized, placebo-controlled study for the treatment of both acne and acne-induced PIH in patients with Fitzpatrick skin types IV–VI.[34] Changes were assessed using a chromameter, PIH severity scale, and Patient's Global Assessment score. The study did not reach statistical significance in measures of efficacy using the assessment scales. The chromameter scores did not show a significant decrease in melanin or erythema during the study; however, the study did not demonstrate an increase in irritation, suggesting clindamycin/tretinoin is nonirritating and well tolerated. Validated outcome measures for PIH would be helpful for similar studies in the future.

Surgical Treatment Options

Laser treatment of PIH has been disappointing and there are very few studies specifically evaluating the use of laser devices in the treatment of PIH for all skin types.[1,3] Although there have been case reports of successful treatment of PIH in darker skin types with blue light phototherapy, fractional thermolysis, and neodymium-doped yttrium aluminum garnet laser, larger clinical studies with validated outcome measures are needed to evaluate their role and efficacy in the treatment of PIH.

Summary/Discussion

- Long-term daily therapy with HQ can result in irritant reactions and exogenous ochronosis
- Use of retinoids can induce retinoid dermatitis in dark-skinned individuals
- Careful selection and caution should be practiced when using a chemical peel to avoid irritation, which can worsen PIH and further complicate management
- Evidence for the various available treatment modalities for PIH is not strong and is underpowered by small population size, poor study design, and validated outcome measures
- Many modalities available for treatment, especially laser therapy, lack proper well-designed, placebo-controlled studies specifically in patients with PIH
- Few studies focus on therapy and outcomes specifically in dark-skinned patients

The use of validated outcome measures in clinical studies investigating the efficacy of therapies available for PIH would further assist in the development of a standardized management for this difficult-to-manage condition. Further research is needed to determine an optimal treatment regimen for PIH, because many of the previously investigated treatment modalities have the potential to exacerbate and worsen inflammation. As evidenced by the studies reviewed, outcomes in novel treatments for PIH remain unsatisfactory.

PHARMACOLOGIC TREATMENT OPTIONS (DPN AND SEBORRHEIC KERATOSIS)

DPN is a benign skin condition characterized by 1- to 5-mm pigmented papules on the face[35] and is considered a variant of seborrheic keratosis (**Fig. 3**). Although the face is the most common location, lesions can appear on the neck, chest, and back as well. This condition is commonly observed individuals of darker skin type, with reported incidence rates of 70% in African Americans and 40% in Asians. Due to the benign nature of this disorder, treatment is not mandatory; however, removal of lesions can be performed to exclude malignancy, for persistent mechanical irritation, inflammation, bleeding, or itching. Most patients are asymptomatic and prefer removal for cosmetic reasons.[36] Previous reports have shown effectiveness of topical vitamin D analogues in the treatment of DPN-type seborrheic keratosis, with application once or twice daily for 3 to 12 months. Only one-third of lesions resolved completely, while other lesions showed a decrease in volume. Tazarotene 0.1% in cream base applied twice daily has also achieved resolution of lesions confirmed by histology, but caused significant irritation.[36] Systemic therapy for multiple seborrheic keratosis would be useful; however, studies using systemic administration of 1,25 dihydroxyvitamin D_3 at 2 high-dose levels led to inflammatory changes of lesions with scarring or brown macules. Thus, topical and systemic therapies have not yet proven to be successful treatment options for seborrheic keratosis (**Fig. 4**).

Surgical Treatment Options

Current treatment options include excision, electrodessication, cryosurgery, curettage, dermabrasion,

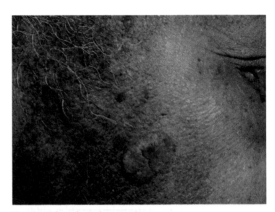

Fig. 4. Seborrheic keratosis.

and laser removal.[35] In a prospective, randomized, controlled, split-face, open-label study comparing electrodessication versus potassium-titanyl phosphate (KTP) laser in 14 African American patients with Fitzpatrick skin types IV–VI with DPN, investigator ratings did not find a statistically significant difference in improvement.[37] Subjects were randomized to receive 2 KTP laser treatments 4 weeks apart to half of the face, and the contralateral side received 2 electrodessication treatments at the same interval time periods. The authors found that KTP treatment was safe and well tolerated, with subjects preferring KTP laser to electrodessication, although this result did not reach statistical significance in subjective discomfort.

A recent trial attempted to determine the comparative efficacy of cryosurgery and curettage in the treatment of seborrheic keratosis.[38] In a 6-week randomized study in 25 adults by Wood and colleagues,[38] 60% of the patients preferred cryotherapy and 36% preferred curettage, with 4% undecided. At 12 months, 61% preferred cryotherapy and 39% preferred curettage. Sixty-four percent of patients preferred cryotherapy over curettage due to decreased postoperative wound care. However, the study did not demonstrate statistically significant differences in subject ratings for cosmetic improvement at either 6-week or 12-month follow-up. Additional studies using standardized techniques, assessment, and different skin types are warranted. Although this study did not compare treatment on facial seborrheic keratosis in dark-skinned patients, further studies investigating their comparative efficacy in this location are recommended.

Pulsed dye laser (PDL) has been used to treat vascular lesions because of its absorption by hemoglobin; however, melanin has also been shown to absorb PDL energy.[39] PDL has been shown to be effective in the treatment of lentigines, ephelides, and seborrheic keratoses. A small

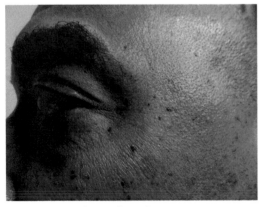

Fig. 3. Dermatosis papulosa nigra.

prospective, controlled, investigator-blinded pilot study compared the efficacy and complications of PDL therapy in 10 patients for the treatment of DPN with curettage and electrodessication. Of the 10 studied subjects, 4 were African American and were followed over a period of at least 12 weeks. The authors found that curettage had the greatest mean percentage clearance (95%),

followed by electrodessication (92.5%) and laser (88%); however, there was no statistical significance in percentage clearance between the 3 modalities ($P = .94$). The study did find a significant difference in subjective pain ratings, patient subjective assessment of cosmetic outcome, and level of posttreatment hyperpigmentation ($P = .12, .34, .61$, respectively). This trial had a

Table 4
Studies evaluating surgical treatment of DPN

Therapy	Treatment	Outcome	Comments
Electrodessication[33]	2 sessions 4 wk apart. Low setting, 0.8 W (range 0.6–1.0 W), treatment to contralateral side of face receiving KTP laser treatment	4% of patients experienced 51%–75% improvement, 4% experienced 1%–25% improvement	Greater discomfort than KTP laser, limitation includes lack of anesthesia
Cryotherapy[34]	Liquid nitrogen in a 1-cycle stutter technique to ensure that the freezing stayed within the confines of lesion and to ensure complete freezing for 12 s, on each side of trunk or proximal extremity. Follow-up at 6 wk and 12 mo after each session	At 6 wk and 12 mo follow-up 60% and 61% of subjects preferred cryotherapy. No statically significant difference reached in subject assessment for improvement of cosmesis	Investigators and participants made assessments subjectively. Limitations include Fitzpatrick skin types I–III only, lack of standardization of cryotherapy technique, varying locations of studied lesions, and age variation in participants
Curettage[34]	4-mm reusable sterile curette, lesion scraped until removed. Lesions were anesthetized before treatment	Increased erythema at 6 wk, formation of hypopigmented scar at 12 wk based on blinded physician postoperative rating scale (2.6 and −0.94, respectively)	
Laser			
KTP[33]	2 sessions 4 wk apart, fluence of 15 J/cm^2, a 10-ms pulse width, 5 pulses per second on a 1-mm spot. Follow-up at 1 mo after last treatment	No statistically significant difference in efficacy vs electrodessication by objective assessment. 21% of patients experienced a 51%–75% improvement	No significant adverse effects, less discomfort reported compared with electrodessication
PDL[39]	7-mm spot size, 10 J/cm^2, and a 10-ms pulse duration; 4 lesions chosen on 10 patients, each to randomly receive PDL, electrodessication, curettage, or control (no treatment). Follow-up at 6 and 12 wk after treatment	No statistically significant difference in percentage of clearance between the 3 treatment modalities	Hyperpigmentation most common adverse outcome in all treatments. Assessments by subjects and investigators were subjective

small sample size, and a larger population may have shown differences in efficacy, patient preference, and adverse events between the 3 modalities (**Table 4**).

Determining which treatment modality is most effective for this common condition should be investigated with larger populations in randomized control trials using objective assessment of discrete lesions with quantifiable measures. Recent studies have failed to show improved efficacy compared with already established treatment modalities. Summarizing the reports above, laser therapy has shown superior efficacy in treatment of DPN and seborrheic keratosis versus topical treatment. No laser therapy has been shown to have greater efficacy in clinical trials compared with standard treatment with electrodessication and curettage, although results are limited due to lack of statistical significance, small population size, and variations in outcome measures.

PHARMACOLOGIC TREATMENT OPTIONS (LICHEN PLANUS PIGMENTOSUS/EDP OF FACE)

EDP, also known as "ashy dermatosis," is commonly seen in dark-skinned patients and is characterized by asymptomatic, slowly progressive, ashy blue-gray macules of the skin.[40,41] The cause of EDP is unknown. It has been suggested to resemble lichen planus pigmentosus (LPP), an immunologically mediated disorder. EDP does not involve mucosal surfaces, whereas LPP does.[9] HQ and tretinoin have been relatively ineffective in the treatment of EDP, as described previously by Stratigos and Katsambas.[1] Dapsone has also been investigated in the treatment of EDP in a small study, demonstrating success and improvement in pigmentation, and complete remission of disease in patients who took the medication at 100 mg/d for 8 to 12 weeks.[40] Clofazamine, which has also been used in the treatment of lupus erythematosus and other

inflammatory dermatosis, showed improvement in a small study with 4 patients after 8 months of treatment at a dose of 100 mg/d.[42] Limitations included characteristic orange-red color of skin induced by treatment, masking improvement of the lesions. Griseofulvin has previously been reported to induce remission, but lesions recur on removal of treatment.[43] Similarly, antibiotics, topical corticosteroids, keratinolytic agents, isoniazid, chloroquine, and psychotherapy have been attempted in treating this disorder, but all demonstrated poor response (**Table 5**).

The treatment of LPP has been a challenge with contemporary treatment modalities proving ineffective (**Fig. 5**).[44] Unfortunately, this disorder is chronic, often persisting for years. Previously, Vitamin A and local and systemic corticosteroids have been shown to help in the clearance of lesions.[44] A recent open-label, nonrandomized, prospective study of topical tacrolimus 0.03% applied twice daily for 6 to 12 weeks reported a 53.8% lightening of pigmentation after treatment in 13 patients.[45] Response to treatment was assessed by grading improvement in pigmentation. Of patients, 57.1% were graded as having excellent improvement and 42.9% were graded as good. Limitations of this study were lack of histologic grading after treatment and small population size. The authors recommended further investigation in a double-blinded manner with a larger number of patients.

Combination Therapies

Other authors have recommended the combination of dapsone and topical tacrolimus along with photoprotection to prevent the progression of LPP.[44]

Surgical Therapies

The efficacy of fractional laser therapy (FLT) in the treatment of EDP and PIH has recently been investigated in a randomized controlled

---

Table 5
Studies evaluating treatment for erythema dyschromicum perstans

Therapy	Treatment	Outcomes
HQ/tretinoin[1]	Dose and duration not specified	Recommendations made by author, not effective
Dapsone[42]	100 mg/d for 8–12 wk	Histologic evaluation of 1 patient before onset of treatment, response measured as complete resolution of lesions
Clofazamine[43]	100 mg/d for 3–8 mo	Cell adhesion molecules ICAM1 and HLA-DR on epidermal keratinocytes disappeared after treatment based on immunohistologic evaluation

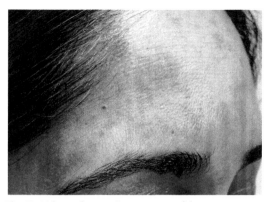

Fig. 5. Lichen planus pigmentosus of face.

observer-blinded study.[46] Patients received 5 nonablative FLT treatments in a 3-week interval between each session, using lower density settings in dark-skinned patients to reduce the risk of developing PIH. Improvement of hyperpigmentation was objectively assessed by reflectance spectroscopy; melanin index was also measured using a DermaSpectrophotometer, and histopathology was used at the 3-month follow-up period. The authors did not find a significant difference in reflectance spectroscopy, melanin index, or histopathology in the amount of dermal melanin after the procedure and thus determined that FLT was not effective for the treatment of EDP. Patients also were unsatisfied with therapy, with most experiencing erythema and a burning sensation.

A consensus on the management of EDP and LPP has not yet been obtained, and although several different treatment modalities have been investigated, most are small or have shown poor response. Further studies using larger population size and methods are required to determine the most effective treatments for this chronic disorder. Although numerous topical therapies have been investigated, results are disappointing, requiring further investigation into developing novel treatments.

REFERENCES

1. Stratigos AJ, Katsambas AD. Optimal management of recalcitrant disorders of hyperpigmentation in dark-skinned patients. Am J Clin Dermatol 2004; 5(3):161–8.
2. Taylor SC. Skin of color: biology, structure, function, and implications for dermatologic disease. J Am Acad Dermatol 2002;46(Suppl 2):S41–62.
3. Davis EC, Callender VD. Postinflammatory hyperpigmentation: a review of the epidemiology, clinical features, and treatment options in skin of color. J Clin Aesthet Dermatol 2010;3(7):20–31.
4. Halder RM, Nootheti PK. Ethnic skin disorders overview. J Am Acad Dermatol 2003;48(Suppl 6): S143–8.
5. Alexis AF, Sergay AB, Taylor SC. Common dermatologic disorders in skin of color: a comparative practice survey. Cutis 2007;80(5):387–94.
6. Sheth VM, Pandya AG. Melasma: a comprehensive update: part I. J Am Acad Dermatol 2011;65(4): 689–97.
7. Kimbrough-Green CK, Griffiths CE, Finkel LJ, et al. Topical retinoic acid (tretinoin) for melasma in black patients. A vehicle-controlled clinical trial. Arch Dermatol 1994;130(6):727–33.
8. Pandya AG, Hynan LS, Bhore R, et al. Reliability assessment and validation of the Melasma Area and Severity Index (MASI) and a new modified MASI scoring method. J Am Acad Dermatol 2011; 64(1):78–83, 83.e1–2.
9. Taylor S, Westerhof W, Im S, et al. Noninvasive techniques for the evaluation of skin color. J Am Acad Dermatol 2006;54(5 Suppl 2):S282–90.
10. Clarys P, Alewaeters K, Lambrecht R, et al. Skin color measurements: comparison between three instruments: the Chromameter(R), the DermaSpectrometer(R) and the Mexameter(R). Skin Res Technol 2000;6(4):230–8.
11. Shriver MD, Parra EJ. Comparison of narrow-band reflectance spectroscopy and tristimulus colorimetry for measurements of skin and hair color in persons of different biological ancestry. Am J Phys Anthropol 2000;112(1):17–27.
12. Lamel SA, Rahvar M, Maibach HI. Postinflammatory hyperpigmentation secondary to external insult: an overview of the quantitative analysis of pigmentation. Cutan Ocul Toxicol 2013;32(1): 67–71.
13. Sheth VM, Pandya AG. Melasma: a comprehensive update: part II. J Am Acad Dermatol 2011;65(4): 699–714.
14. Sarkar R, Kaur C, Bhalla M, et al. The combination of glycolic acid peels with a topical regimen in the treatment of melasma in dark-skinned patients: a comparative study. Dermatol Surg 2002;28(9): 828–32.
15. Erbil H, Sezer E, Taştan B, et al. Efficacy and safety of serial glycolic acid peels and a topical regimen in the treatment of recalcitrant melasma. J Dermatol 2007;34(1):25–30.
16. Grimes P, Kelly AP, Torok H, et al. Community-based trial of a triple-combination agent for the treatment of facial melasma. Cutis 2006;77(3):177–84.
17. Guevara IL, Pandya AG. Melasma treated with hydroquinone, tretinoin, and a fluorinated steroid. Int J Dermatol 2001;40(3):212–5.
18. Goldberg DJ, Berlin AL, Phelps R. Histologic and ultrastructural analysis of melasma after fractional resurfacing. Lasers Surg Med 2008;40(2):134–8.

19. Karsai S, Fischer T, Pohl L, et al. Is non-ablative 1550-nm fractional photothermolysis an effective modality to treat melasma? Results from a prospective controlled single-blinded trial in 51 patients. J Eur Acad Dermatol Venereol 2012;26(4): 470–6.

20. Li YH, Chen JZ, Wei HC, et al. Efficacy and safety of intense pulsed light in treatment of melasma in Chinese patients. Dermatol Surg 2008;34(5): 693–700.

21. Wang CC, Hui CY, Sue YM, et al. Intense pulsed light for the treatment of refractory melasma in Asian persons. Dermatol Surg 2004;30(9):1196–200.

22. Sivayathorn A, Verallo-Rowell V, Graupe K. 20% azelaic acid cream in the topical treatment of melasma: a double-blind comparison with 2% hydroquinone. Eur J Dermatol 1995;5:680–4.

23. Espinal-Pérez LE, Moncada B, Castañedo-cazares JP. A double-blind randomized trial of 5% ascorbic acid vs. 4% hydroquinone in melasma. Int J Dermatol 2004;43(8):604–7.

24. Lim JT. Treatment of melasma using kojic acid in a gel containing hydroquinone and glycolic acid. Dermatol Surg 1999;25(4):282–4.

25. Savory S, Agim NG, Pandya AG, et al. Reliability assessment and validation of the postacne hyperpigmentation index (PAHPI), a new instrument to measure postinflammatory hyperpigmentation from acne vulgaris. J Am Acad Dermatol 2014;70(1): 108–14. http://dx.doi.org/10.1016/j.jaad.2013.09.017.

26. Taylor SC, Callender VD. A multicenter, 12-week, phase 3b trial: a combination solution of mequinol 2%/tretinoin 0.01% vs. hydroquinone 4% cream in the treatment of mild to moderate postinflammatory hyperpigmentation [abstract]. J Am Acad Dermatol 2006;54(Suppl):AB194.

27. Bulengo-Ransby SM, Griffiths CE, Kimbrough-Green CK, et al. Topical tretinoin (retinoic acid) therapy for hyperpigmented lesions caused by inflammation of the skin in black patients. N Engl J Med 1993;328(20):1438–43.

28. Grimes P, Callender V. Tazarotene cream for postinflammatory hyperpigmentation and acne vulgaris in darker skin: a double-blind, randomized, vehicle-controlled study. Cutis 2006;77(1): 45–50.

29. Lee DH, Oh IY, Koo KT, et al. Reduction in facial hyperpigmentation after treatment with a combination of topical niacinamide and tranexamic acid: a randomized, double-blind, vehicle-controlled trial. Skin Res Technol 2013;0:1–5.

30. Grimes PE. Management of hyperpigmentation in darker racial ethnic groups. Semin Cutan Med Surg 2009;28(2):77–85.

31. Burns RL, Prevost-blank PL, Lawry MA, et al. Glycolic acid peels for postinflammatory hyperpigmentation in black patients. A comparative study. Dermatol Surg 1997;23(3):171–4.

32. Academy Issues updated position statement on vitamin D. Available at: http://www.aad.org/stories-and-news/news-releases/academy-issues-updated-position-statement-on-vitamin-d. Accessed September 27, 2013.

33. Kato H, Araki J, Eto H, et al. A prospective randomized controlled study of oral tranexamic acid for preventing postinflammatory hyperpigmentation after Q-switched ruby laser. Dermatol Surg 2011;37(5): 605–10.

34. Callender VD, Young CM, Kindred C, et al. Efficacy and safety of clindamycin phosphate 1.2% and tretinoin 0.025% gel for the treatment of acne and acne-induced post-inflammatory hyperpigmentation in patients with skin of color. J Clin Aesthet Dermatol 2012;5(7):25–32.

35. Taylor SC, Averyhart AN, Heath CR. Postprocedural wound-healing efficacy following removal of dermatosis papulosa nigra lesions in an African American population: a comparison of a skin protectant ointment and a topical antibiotic. J Am Acad Dermatol 2011;64(Suppl 3):S30–5.

36. Hafner C, Vogt T. Seborrheic keratosis. J Dtsch Dermatol Ges 2008;6(8):664–77.

37. Kundu RV, Joshi SS, Suh KY, et al. Comparison of electrodessication and potassium-titanyl-phosphate laser for treatment of dermatosispapulosanigra. Dermatol Surg 2009;35(7):1079–83.

38. Wood LD, Stucki JK, Hollenbeak CS, et al. Effectiveness of cryosurgery vs. curettage in the treatment of seborrheic keratoses. JAMA Dermatol 2013;149(1): 108–9.

39. Garcia MS, Azari R, Eisen DB. Treatment of dermatosis papulosa nigra in 10 patients: a comparison trial of electrodessication, pulsed dye laser, and curettage. Dermatol Surg 2010;36(12):1968–72.

40. Bahadir S, Cobanoglu U, Cimsit G, et al. Erythema dyschromicum perstans: response to dapsone therapy. Int J Dermatol 2004;43(3):220–2.

41. Schwartz RA. Erythema dyschromicum perstans: the continuing enigma of Cinderella or ashy dermatosis. Int J Dermatol 2004;43(3):230–2.

42. Barranda L, Torres-Alvarez B, Cortes-Franco R, et al. Involvement of cell adhesion and activation molecules in the pathogenesis of erythema dyschromicum perstans (ashy dermatitis). The effect of clofazamine therapy. Arch Dermatol 1997;133(3): 325–9.

43. Kontochristopolus G, Stavropoulus P, Panteleos D, et al. Erythema dyschromicum perstans: response to dapsone therapy. Int J Dermatol 1998;37: 790–9.

44. Sehgal VN, Verma P, Bhattacharya SN, et al. Lichen planus pigmentosus. Skinmed 2013;11(2): 96–103.

45. Al-Mutairi N, El-khalawany M. Clinicopathological characteristics of lichen planus pigmentosus and its response to tacrolimus ointment: an open label, non-randomized, prospective study. J Eur Acad Dermatol Venereol 2010;24(5):535–40.

46. Kroon MW, Wind BS, Meesters AA, et al. Non-ablative 1550 nm fractional laser therapy not effective for erythema dyschromicum perstans and postinflammatory hyperpigmentation: a pilot study. J Dermatolog Treat 2012;23(5):339–44.

Cosmeceuticals
Efficacy and Influence on Skin Tone

Zoe Diana Draelos, MD*

KEYWORDS

- Cosmeceuticals • Skin tone • Postinflammatory hyperpigmentation • Topical formulations
- Dyspigmentation

KEY POINTS

- Cosmeceuticals form an important part of the over-the-counter skin treatment market, especially in persons of African descent.
- Some industry forecasters believe that the cosmetics industry has hit a glass ceiling in new cosmeceutical development, largely because of the failure of the US Food and Drug Administration to develop a new classification system.
- It is believed that a new quasidrug category, similar to the Japanese designation, would allow the introduction of more robust active ingredients into cosmeceuticals.
- Although claims are made for various cosmetic ingredients such as vitamin C and E, there is a lack of scientific evidence of their efficacy.
- Dermatology will move the cosmeceutical category forward, and the cosmeceutical category will move dermatology forward.

INTRODUCTION
Cosmeceuticals and the Regulatory Environment

Cosmeceuticals, from a consumer standpoint, are believed to be a category of skin care products that function as active cosmetics going beyond mere adornment and scenting of the skin. Yet, from a regulatory standpoint, cosmeceuticals is an unrecognized term with no meaning, because cosmeceuticals are purely cosmetics and viewed as such in the United States.[1] In dermatology, cosmeceuticals are believed to encompass the topical application of biologically active ingredients, which affect the skin barrier and overall skin health.[2] The ability of cosmeceuticals to enhance skin functioning depends on the incorporation of ingredients into a topical vehicle that maintains the integrity of the active, delivers the active in a biologically appropriate form, reaches the target site in sufficient quantity to exert an effect, and properly releases the ingredient from the carrier vehicle. Clinical testing using the scientific method for efficacy assessment must be performed to document the value of the cosmeceutical.

Because cosmeceuticals are considered cosmetics, safety to the consumer is of key importance. Most cosmeceuticals are formulated from ingredients that already have a proven safety record in the marketplace. This situation may be because of their extraction from foods, such as topical lycopene from tomatoes or topical avocadin from avocados. Alternatively, extensive animal testing may be undertaken by the raw material supplier to determine that the new ingredient is appropriate for human use. In the case of botanicals, most are assumed safe based on their ubiquitous nature. To avoid regulatory issues, most cosmeceuticals use ingredients that are generally recognized as safe, which is how cosmetics are also formulated.

No relevant conflicts of interest.
Department of Dermatology, Duke University School of Medicine, Durham, NC, USA
* 2444 North Main Street, High Point, NC 27262.
E-mail address: zdraelos@northstate.net

Dermatol Clin 32 (2014) 137–143
http://dx.doi.org/10.1016/j.det.2013.12.002
0733-8635/14/$ – see front matter © 2014 Elsevier Inc. All rights reserved.

This article discusses cosmeceuticals and their efficacy. It examines available testing methodologies used to better understand how cosmeceuticals affect the skin and the various mechanisms of action cosmeceuticals use to improve skin appearance. The discussion focuses on skin tone and what this term means in persons of African descent and how problems can be avoided when using cosmeceuticals in skin of color.

Development of Scientific Substantiation

Cosmeceutical formulations must be tested for 3 important reasons: (1) to determine that they provide a benefit that is perceived by the consumer; (2) to establish that the formulation is safe and free of adverse reactions; and (3) to support marketing claims. Consumers purchase a new cosmeceutical once based on the name, promises made on the packaging, recommendations from advertising or acquaintances, appearance, and fragrance. However, the consumer does not re-purchase a product that is not perceived to work. In many regards, the consumer is the most discriminating grader when it comes to cosmeceutical preparations. Most cosmetic companies carry out extensive consumer testing before a product is released into the marketplace. This testing is then backed up by dermatologist-led testing to determine efficacy but also to ensure that the product does not cause any adverse reactions, such as allergic contact dermatitis, irritant contact dermatitis, comedogenicity, or acnegenicity.[3] Testing is sometimes performed in conjunction with an ophthalmologist to ensure that no eye issues arise as a result of accidental eye instillation.

In addition to clinical testing to assess consumer subjective evaluations and dermatologist objective evaluations, noninvasive testing is also performed to confirm the visual and tactile observations. Noninvasive testing is used because it does not enter the body and evaluates skin performance by placing electronic sensors or devices on the skin to gain insight into skin functioning. This type of testing allows product evaluation without the traditional biopsy that is used for medical diagnostic purposes. If a cosmeceutical manufacturer made claims based on biopsy information, such as "this cream increases type III collagen production," it could be considered a drug. Noninvasive testing avoids this conundrum and allows efficacy evaluations in a scientific manner without entering the skin.

The need for scientific substantiation of cosmeceutical performance has led to the development of skin bioengineering. Skin bioengineering develops equipment to assess skin functioning before and after product application to detect small changes that might not be visually or tactilely perceived (**Box 1**). Sometimes, clinical studies must be run in 4 to 12 weeks for practical reasons, and it is hoped that small skin improvements might become magnified over time with continued use. Usually, noninvasive results parallel clinical results in an efficacious formulation.

The most common claim for substantiation in cosmeceuticals is skin moisturization. Moisturization can decrease fine lines of dehydration, improve skin smoothness, decrease itching, and increase light reflection from the skin surface. All of these benefits enhance the visual, tactile, and sensory functioning of the skin. Corneometry is the technique used to determine how much water is present in the skin, which is one way of assessing skin moisturization. Corneometry uses a probe that emits and receives low current electricity. The electrical current is transmitted into the skin by the sending portion of the probe and received. This measure is an indication of the electrical conductivity of the skin. Because water is an excellent conductor of electricity, skin water content can be measured. More water in the skin correlates with better skin appearance and functioning, translated to the consumer as better skin moisturization. Thus, corneometry is the noninvasive bioengineering assessment technique used to substantiate claims of enhanced skin moisturization.

Moisturization can also be evaluated by assessing the integrity of the skin barrier. An intact skin barrier prevents water loss and encourages superior skin moisturization, whereas a damaged barrier encourages transepidermal water loss. The noninvasive test to measure transepidermal water loss is evaporimetry.[4] Evaporimetry uses a probe that senses the humidity of the air directly above the skin. The probe contains 2 humidity meters, which are placed at known distances above the skin. The water vapor passes between the 2 fixed distance humidity meters through an orifice of

---

Box 1
Bioengineering tests relevant to cosmeceutical testing

a. Corneometry

b. Evaporimetry

c. Silicone replicas

d. Chromametry

e. Laser Doppler flowmetry

known diameter. The difference in the observed humidity between the 2 meters is calculated. By comparing the amount of water leaving the skin before and after cosmeceutical moisturizer application, the effect of the moisturization on skin hydration can be determined. Quality moisturizers decrease transepidermal water loss in barrier-damaged skin.[5] It is through the use of corneometry and evaporimetry that claims of "45% increase in moisturization in 10 minutes" can be substantiated.

Noninvasive techniques can also be used to assess the improvement in fine lines and wrinkles. This technique is known as profilometry. Profilometry uses unpolymerized silicone, in the form of dental impression material, which is mixed with a catalyst just before skin application. The polymerizing silicone is placed in a round form on the face, usually around the lateral eye, to capture wrinkling in the crow's feet area. This area of the eye is used because it is the thinnest skin on the body commonly affected by dehydration, which is easiest to improve texturally with moisturizers. As the silicone polymerizes on the skin, a replica is obtained of the skin topography. The replica is a negative of the skin dermatoglyphics, showing mountains for depressed wrinkles and valleys where the skin surface is smooth.[6]

Replicas are allowed to cure for 24 hours and then analyzed with a scanning laser to determine the depth, number, and contour of the wrinkles. Computer imaging can transform the scan into a two-dimensional or three-dimensional topogram, which can be used in advertising and on packaging to convince consumers of the capability of the moisturizer to reduce fine lines. Scientifically, before and after replicas are compared to determine the effect of the moisturizer on skin fine lines and wrinkles. This is the method used to substantiate claims of "56% fine line reduction in 5 days."

Bioengineering methods can also be used to assess color changes in the skin through techniques known as chromametry and Doppler flowmetry. Chromametry uses a colorimeter, originally developed to match paint colors, to evaluate the color of the skin on 3 axes known as L, a, and b.[7] The colorimeter can give readings to assess skin color changes in terms of all hues, but usually brown and red pigmentation are assessed.[8] Claims of improved skin color, radiance, and luminosity can be substantiated through chromametry.

Skin redness can also be measured in terms of blood flow alterations with a technique known as laser Doppler flowmetry.[9] This technique makes use of the Doppler effect to measure the speed of blood flow in the skin. Enhanced blood flow equates with increased skin redness. Although adequate blood flow is necessary to have pink healthy skin, too much blood flow indicates inflammation and equates with the red face of dermatologic disease. However, increased blood can minimize the sallow appearance of photodamaged skin. A few cosmeceuticals contain botanic vasodilators to improve skin color and substantiate these claims using flowmetry.

All of the noninvasive techniques previously discussed are used to add further information to subjective patient assessments and visual trained observer assessments. They are not a substitute for good clinical testing. The human eye is still the best measure of cosmeceutical efficacy. Most cosmeceutical claims are based on the evaluations of the subject and the investigator, which are accurate if the study is a well-designed double-blind vehicle-controlled trial.

Cosmeceutical Development

Many ingredients are derived from a variety of different sources that are used in cosmeceutical formulations. The possibilities are endless, given the sophistication of the plant kingdom, providing more variety than is currently available in pharmaceuticals. The development process for new cosmeceutical ingredients combines exploration with analytical chemistry with sophisticated gene chip arrays, cell culture models, animal studies, and human trials, similar to the methodology used to develop new pharmaceuticals. The only missing piece of information is the dose, because cosmeceuticals are not intended for ingestion. The cosmeceutical development process is summarized in **Box 2**.

Cosmeceutical Claims

Cosmeceuticals are defined by the claims that are made regarding their intended use. A product that eliminates wrinkles is a drug, whereas a product that minimizes the appearance of wrinkles is a cosmetic, even although they may both contain the same ingredients. It seems unscientific to define product functioning based on package labeling and advertising, yet this is our current level of sophistication. Cosmeceuticals that function too well would alter the structure and function of the skin and become drugs. The current state of the cosmeceutical marketplace is not a result of the industry's lack of desire to perform thoughtful research and develop quality products but rather a result of limitations imposed by the present regulatory climate regarding product claims. Thus, cosmeceuticals are cosmetics and only appearance claims can be made rather than functional claims.

Mechanism of Action for Cosmeceuticals

Currently marketed cosmeceuticals provide skin benefits through a few well-established mechanisms of action. The two of primary importance are barrier enhancement and photoprotection. These are activities that modify the stratum corneum, which is nonliving, and clearly fall within the intended cosmetic realm. The remainder of the cosmeceutical functional categories alter the structure and function of the skin, making them drugs and not cosmetics. Yet, there are products in the marketplace that contain ingredients functioning through these mechanisms, but the claims made are appearance claims and not functional claims, allowing them to be sold as cosmeceuticals.

Barrier function
The main cutaneous function of cosmeceuticals is to enhance the barrier function of the skin. Enhancing the barrier decreases stinging and burning from a sensory standpoint and improves the look and feel of the skin. Moisturizers are the main cosmeceutical category, which smooth down desquamating corneocytes and fill in the gaps between the remaining corneocytes to create the impression of tactile smoothness. This effect is temporary, of course, until the moisturizer is removed from the skin surface by wiping or cleansing. This factor allows moisturizers to be considered cosmetics. From a functional standpoint, moisturizers can create an optimal environment for healing and minimize the appearance of lines of dehydration by decreasing transepidermal water loss. Transepidermal water loss increases when the brick and mortar organization of the protein-rich corneocytes held together by intercellular lipids is damaged. A well-formulated cosmeceutical moisturizer can decrease water loss until healing occurs, which is definitely a functional effect on the skin. Thus, cosmeceutical moisturizers can improve the appearance of dry skin, but not treat eczema.

Photoprotection
In addition to providing moisturization benefits, many cosmeceuticals make antiaging claims based on the presence of a sunscreen ingredient. The new sunscreen guidance allows antiaging claims on sunscreen-containing products based on the inclusion of ingredients from the US Sunscreen Monograph. This regulatory change is based on the recognition that sunscreens promote younger-looking skin that is less photoaged.

Many new developments have occurred in the photoprotection cosmeceutical market to increase both efficacy and cosmetic acceptability. Higher sun protection factor (SPF) formulations are more popular as new sunscreen combinations arise that provide better UV-B protection. New methods of increasing the longevity of UV-A photoprotectants provide better broad-spectrum protection. Dry touch sunscreens have even been developed that dry quickly in place on the skin surface, preventing rub-off and a sticky feel. All of these advances make sunscreens able to provide superior photoprotection.

Pigment lightening
Facial hyperpigmentation is one of the most common signs of photoaging. Many different patterns can be seen. Focal hyperpigmentation in the form of small lentigines across the lateral cheeks usually begins about age 25 to 30 years, depending on cumulative sun exposure, with continued accumulation of lesions throughout life. Pigmentation can also present in the form of melasma, with reticulated pigment over the sides of the forehead lateral jawline and upper lip. Hyperpigmentation can present as overall darkening of the skin from a combination of melanin pigment, fragmented elastin fibers, and residual hemosiderin. Cosmeceutical treatments for hyperpigmentation are

becoming more numerous as the safety of prescription hydroquinone is challenged by regulatory bodies worldwide.

Receptor activation

The next important mechanism of action for cosmeceuticals is receptor activation. There is only 1 skin receptor that has been well characterized: the retinoid receptor.[10] Prescription retinoids, such as tazarotene and tretinoin, are well studied for their ability to induce profound skin changes; however, over-the-counter (OTC) retinoids may show some of the same effects, to a lesser degree.[11,12] It is theoretically possible to interconvert the retinoids from 1 form to another. For example, retinyl palmitate and retinyl propionate, chemically known as retinyl esters, can become biologically active after cutaneous enzymatic cleavage of the ester bond and subsequent conversion to retinol. Retinol is the naturally occurring vitamin A form found in red, yellow, and orange fruits and vegetables. Retinol can be oxidized to retinaldehyde and then oxidized to retinoic acid, also known as prescription tretinoin. It is this cutaneous conversion of retinol to retinoic acid that is responsible for the biological activity of some of the new stabilized OTC vitamin A preparations designed to improve the appearance of benign photodamaged skin.[13] Only small amounts of retinyl palmitate and retinol can be converted by the skin, yet retinoid receptor activation by retinol remains one of the best understood cosmeceutical mechanisms of action.

Peptide cellular messengers

Peptides as modulators of cellular communication are one of the newest cosmetic ingredient mechanisms of action. Peptides are the building blocks of proteins, and proteins have been used for many years in cosmetics. Proteins, obtained from boiled cow skin, are used as thickeners and humectants. However, the use of engineered proteins with biological activity is novel. Because the body uses peptides to communicate between cells, it was theorized that perhaps engineered peptides might be able to upregulate or downregulate cutaneous functions. The upregulation or downregulation of cellular factors is definitely in the drug realm, but functional claims are not made when peptides are incorporated into cosmeceuticals. This situation may be because it is challenging for peptides to penetrate the skin, and most of the peptide functional research is performed in cell culture.

Antioxidants

Antioxidants form one of the most popular categories of cosmeceutical ingredients. The primary source of cosmeceutical antioxidants is botanic extracts, because all plants must protect themselves from oxidation after ultraviolet (UV) exposure in the outdoor environment in which they grow. Antioxidant botanicals function by quenching singlet oxygen and reactive oxygen species, such as superoxide anions, hydroxyl radicals, fatty peroxy radicals, and hydroperoxides. There are many botanic antioxidants available from raw material suppliers to the cosmeceutical industry, which can be classified into 1 of 3 categories as flavonoids, carotenoids, and polyphenols. Flavonoids possess a polyphenolic structure that accounts for their antioxidant, UV protectant, and metal chelation abilities. Carotenoids are chemically related to retinoids, previously discussed. Polyphenols comprise the largest category of botanic antioxidants. When antioxidants are included in cosmeceutical formulations, claims are made only about their inclusion in the formulation, not about their functionality.

Cosmeceuticals and Skin Tone

The general public perceive cosmeceuticals as creams and lotions that can magically improve the appearance, feel, and condition of their skin. Some even believe that cosmeceuticals can turn back the effects of excessive sun exposure and photoaging. Much of this belief accounts for the hope in the jar opinions that many dermatologists have regarding cosmeceuticals. True efficacy must be separated from marketing gibberish to accurately evaluate this category. It is hoped that this article clarifies some of the issues. Improper use of cosmeceuticals can cause problems, especially in persons of African descent. The rest of this article focuses on cosmeceuticals and their ability to alter skin tone. Although skin tone is a cosmetic term without scientific meaning, skin tone is generally used to denote skin color in combination with skin firmness.

The most popular cosmeceuticals used by persons of African descent are aimed at improving skin pigmentation. Many OTC products contain 2% hydroquinone, which can be a cutaneous irritation. Other pigment-lightening products may contain glycolic or salicylic acid and are intended to improve pigmentation temporarily by inducing exfoliation of the pigmented corneocytes. These low pH ingredients can further irritate the skin, resulting in postinflammatory hyperpigmentation. Skin irritation only darkens skin of African descent; it does not produce the intended lightening.

Other popular cosmeceuticals are cleansers designed to improve skin pigmentation. Many of these products combine surfactants with particulate scrubs, such as nut pits or polyethylene scrubbing beads. The idea is to scrub away the abnormal pigmentation. These products again can cause skin irritation by damaging the stratum corneum and viable epidermis, causing increased rather than decreased pigmentation in persons of African descent. Other scrubbing devices, such at home dermabrasion machines, aggressive mechanized facial brushes, and needling devices, should also be avoided, because they may induce postinflammatory hyperpigmentation.

Persons of African descent should focus on the use of sunscreen-containing moisturizers, which decrease transepidermal water loss, minimize barrier damage, and provide photoprotection. Sunscreen-containing moisturizer should be selected with a minimum SPF 30, because lower SPF products may not have adequate UV-A photoprotection, which is the action spectra for facial pigmentation. Ideally, the sunscreen-containing moisturizer should combine both organic and inorganic filters to both absorb and reflect UV radiation. The moisturizer improves skin firmness by increasing skin water content, and the sunscreen prevents dyspigmentation, resulting in a net improvement in skin tone.

Further photoprotection in persons of African descent can be achieved by applying a facial foundation. Colored cosmetics can be an excellent source of photoprotection. Facial foundation contains iron oxide, zinc oxide, and kaolin, all of which can provide physical broad-spectrum photoprotection. Many facial foundations now contain organic and inorganic sunscreens.

SUMMARY: THE FUTURE

Cosmeceuticals form an important part of the OTC skin treatment market, especially in persons of African descent. Some industry forecasters believe that the cosmetics industry has hit a glass ceiling in new cosmeceutical development, largely because of the failure of the US Food and Drug Administration to develop a new classification system. It is believed that a new quasidrug category, similar to the Japanese designation, would allow the introduction of more robust active ingredients into cosmeceuticals. These more robust ingredients would provide enhanced consumer perceived skin benefits, supporting stronger claims.

Perhaps the most disturbing part of the cosmeceutical category issue is the definition of a dermatologic drug as something that alters the structure and function of the skin. This was the language used in the original Cosmetics and Toiletries Act. The act was written at a time when the skin was believed to be nothing more than a covering on the outside of the body, with little biological activity. We now know that the skin is enzymatically and immunologically active, participating in important metabolic functions required to sustain life. We know that many externally applied substances profoundly influence the skin. Further, although claims are made for various cosmetic ingredients such as vitamin C and E, there is a lack of scientific evidence of their efficacy.

I believe that cosmeceuticals will become an ever-increasing part of the fund of knowledge of dermatology. We are now only at the beginning of the cosmeceutical story. Cosmeceuticals were derived from the cosmetics industry's desire to go beyond simply adorning the skin. The industry wanted to improve the appearance of the skin by tackling important functional issues to meet the demands of all consumers, including those of African descent. Dermatology will move the cosmeceutical category forward, and the cosmeceutical category will move dermatology forward.

REFERENCES

1. Kligman AM. Cosmeceuticals as a third category. Cosmet Toilet 1998;113:33.
2. Vermeer BJ, Gilchrest BA. Cosmeceuticals. A proposal for rational definition, evaluation and regulation. Arch Dermatol 1996;132:337.
3. Jackson EM. Hypoallergenic claims. Am J Contact Dermatitis 1993;4(2):108–10.
4. Agner T, Serup J. Individual and instrumental variations in irritant patch-test reactions: clinical evaluation and quantification by bioengineering methods. Clin Exp Dermatol 1990;15(1):29–33.
5. Idson B. In vivo measurement of transdermal water loss. J Soc Cosmet Chem 1976;29:573–80.
6. Grove GL, Grove MJ. Objective methods for assessing skin surface topography noninvasively. In: Leveque JL, editor. Cutaneous investigation in health and disease. New York: Marcel Dekker; 1988. p. 1–32.
7. Pierard GE, Nikkels AF. Rating sensitive skin by colorimetry of the skin and of D-squame collections. International symposium on irritant contact dermatitis. Groningen, Holland, October 1991.
8. Babulak SW, Rhein LD, Scala DD, et al. Quantification of erythema in a soap chamber test using the Minolta Chroma (Reflectance) Meter. J Soc Cosmet Chem 1986;37:475–9.
9. Nilsson GE, Otto U, Wahlberg JE. Assessment of skin irritancy in man by laser Doppler flowmetry. Contact Dermatitis 1982;8:401–6.
10. Kligman LH, Do CH, Kligman AM. Topical retinoic acid enhances the repair of ultraviolet damaged dermal connective tissue. Connect Tissue Res 1984;12:139–50.

11. Goodman DS. Vitamin A and retinoids in health and disease. N Engl J Med 1984;310(16):1023–31.

12. Noy N. Interactions of retinoids with lipid bilayers and with membranes. In: Livrea MA, Packer L, editors. Retinoids. New York: Marcel Dekker; 1993. p. 17–27.

13. Duell EA, Derguini F, Kang S, et al. Extraction of human epidermis treated with retinol yields retro-retinoids in addition to free retinol and retinyl esters. J Invest Dermatol 1996;107: 178–82.

A Systematic Approach to Afro-Textured Hair Disorders
Dermatoscopy and When to Biopsy

Natalie C. Yin, MD, Antonella Tosti, MD*

KEYWORDS

- Corkscrew hair • Central centrifugal cicatricial alopecia • Dissecting cellulitis
- Frontal fibrosing alopecia • Lichen planopilaris • Alopecia areata • Androgenetic alopecia
- Pinpoint white dots

KEY POINTS

- Trichoscopy of Afro-textured hair and scalp is still evolving.
- Pinpoint white dots are a unique dermoscopic feature of the scalp in people of African ancestry and make diagnosis of scarring alopecia more difficult.
- Dermoscopy is useful in selecting the biopsy site and, ultimately, in increasing the rate of pathologic diagnosis.

INTRODUCTION

Dermatoscopy is a noninvasive technique that has gained wide use in "in vivo" diagnosis of hair diseases. Hair dermatoscopy, also referred to as trichoscopy, facilitates visualization and analysis of scalp and hair structures and patterns. These structures include hair shafts, follicular openings, cutaneous vascular patterns, and perifollicular signs. Given the variation in reproducibility of current diagnostic standards (eg, clinical examination, pull test, and biopsy), trichoscopy serves to improve diagnostic accuracy.[1,2] The extensive study and use in the white population has made it an integral technique used in daily dermatologic practice.

However, to date, little has been published regarding the dermatoscopic findings in hair disorders of Afro-textured hair. Although many of the same diseases affect all hair types, the distinct properties of the hair and scalp in patients of African descent warrant further investigation into the trichoscopic patterns unique to this population. For example, the hair shaft in African American patients is tightly curled in tertiary structure. In cross-section, it is flattened or elliptical.[3] It is common to observe knots and areas of breakage along the hair shaft, which can be easily visualized with the dermatoscope (**Fig. 1**). The hair follicles are similarly curved.[4] Less moisture is also characteristic of hair shafts in African American patients compared with whites.[5] Moreover, the scalp is often more darkly pigmented. This article reviews the current knowledge regarding dermatoscopic findings specific to Afro-textured hair and suggests when trichoscopy-guided biopsy may be appropriate in affected individuals.

NORMAL SCALP

Scalp color in dark-skinned individuals can vary from light brown to dark black on dermatoscopy but does not necessarily correlate with the actual color of the skin. Another typical feature is a

Department of Dermatology and Cutaneous Surgery, University of Miami Miller School of Medicine, 1600 North West 10th Avenue, RMSB, Room 2023-A, Miami, FL 33136, USA
* Corresponding author.
E-mail address: Atosti@med.miami.edu

Dermatol Clin 32 (2014) 145–151
http://dx.doi.org/10.1016/j.det.2013.11.005
0733-8635/14/$ – see front matter © 2014 Elsevier Inc. All rights reserved.

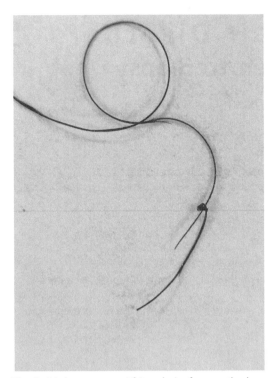

Fig. 1. At dermoscopy, African hairs frequently show knots and fissures.

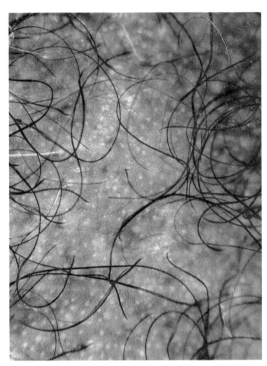

Fig. 2. Pinpoint white dots: dots correspond to follicular and sweat gland openings.

perifollicular pigmented network or honeycomb pattern.[6] The presence of rete ridge melanocytes account for the hyperchromic lines of this pattern, whereas the hypochromic areas have fewer melanocytes residing in the suprapapillary epidermis.[7] Hair density is significantly lower than in white patients (about 18 terminal and 3 vellus hairs in a 4 mm punch) but the hair diameter is larger.[8]

Each follicle contains one or two vellus hairs and between two and four terminal hairs.[6] In general, the hairs display a coarser, curlier texture.[9] A characteristic feature of the pigmented scalp is the presence of small white dots, which have been named pinpoint white dots.[10] Pinpoint white dots appear as small, 0.2 to 0.3 mm, white dots distributed regularly between the follicles among the pigment network (**Fig. 2**).[10] These white dots were originally described by Kossard and Zagarella[7] in the scalp a patient with lichen planopilaris (LPP), but they were misinterpreted as a sign of fibrosis. Abraham and colleagues[11] coined the term pinpoint white dots. They correlated this dermoscopic feature with the opening of the sweat ducts. More recently, reflectance confocal microscopy showed that the pinpoint white dots correspond to acrosyringeal and follicular openings.[12] Pinpoint white dots make distinguishing scarring from nonscarring alopecia more difficult than in

the nonpigmented scalp because the loss of follicular openings is not immediately evident. Scaling is often a prominent feature, possibly related to the high prevalence of seborrheic dermatitis in this population. Vessels are often visible but there are no studies describing the vascular patterns of the normal black scalp.

TINEA CAPITIS

Tinea capitis (TC) is a common dermatophyte infection affecting children, particularly those of African descent. The most commonly reported dermatoscopic findings associated with TC in black children are corkscrew hairs.[13] These were first described by Hughes and colleagues[13] in African children with endothrix TC, particularly of the *Trichophyton soudanense* type. Since then, corkscrew hairs have also been found in TC caused by *T violaceum*.[14] In fact, Vazquez-Lopez and colleagues[14] documented the resolution of corkscrew hairs in TC of an African American child following administration of griseofulvin therapy. These broken, twisted hairs are usually seen in association with comma hairs, which are typically seen in TC of black and white patients (**Fig. 3**). Comma hairs, originally described by Slowinska and colleagues[15] in patients with *Microsporum canis* infection are broken, comma-shaped hairs

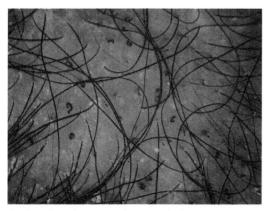

Fig. 3. TC: corkscrew and comma hairs.

that can easily be distinguished from the blunt-ended, tapering hair shaft, exclamation mark hairs in alopecia areata. The comma shape is thought to result from hair shaft cracking and bending because of ectothrix or endothrix fungal infection.[15] Corkscrew hairs are exclusive to African descent patients, in whom they are seen in endothrix and ectothrix infections. Broken hairs and black dots are also observed.[13] The cause for corkscrew hairs is unknown; however, it is likely linked to the anatomic shape of African hairs. Furthermore, the coiled hairs have been found to have many more fungal elements compared to the straight hairs.[16]

ALOPECIA AREATA

Alopecia areata is a common, nonscarring, hair loss disorder. It occurs in whites and African Americans with equal frequency. Despite its prevalence, however, only one study has described the dermatoscopic findings seen in an African American patient.[17] As in normal scalp, the honeycomb-like network can be seen in alopecic patches. Yellow dots are usually absent and the alopecic area shows an increased number of pinpoint white dots. Diagnosis is based on presence of exclamation mark hairs, broken hairs, and black dots (**Fig. 4**).

ALOPECIA DUE TO HAIR BREAKAGE

Hair breakage is common because of the intrinsic characteristics of African hair and the hair shaft damage caused by multiple styling processes. Severe hair breakage, predominantly caused by chemical procedures can cause alopecic patches. Patients complain that their hair does not grow and present a positive tug sign. Dermoscopy is helpful to show breakage with *Trichorrhexis nodosa*, which can be seen in the scalp or, even more easily, in the shed broken hairs (**Fig. 5**).[18]

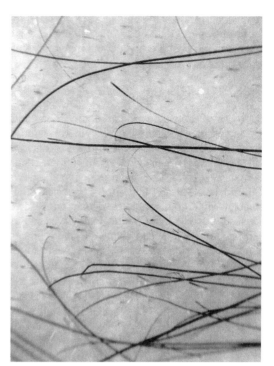

Fig. 4. Alopecia areata: pinpoint white dots, broken hairs, and exclamation mark hairs.

ANDROGENETIC ALOPECIA

In the authors' experience, diagnosis of androgenetic alopecia is difficult in women of African descent, possibly due to its overlap with central

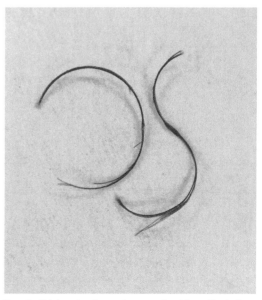

Fig. 5. *Trichorrhexis nodosa* and trichoptilosis in a broken shaft.

centrifugal cicatricial alopecia (CCCA). Dermoscopy shows more than 20% hair shaft variability and presence of short, thin (0.03 mm in diameter) regrowing hairs in the frontal scalp.

CCCA

CCCA is a persistent inflammatory condition, most commonly seen in women of African descent.[19] CCCA is among the top five reasons for dermatologic evaluation in African American women.[20,21] In CCCA, the dermoscopy shows reduced hair density, hair shaft variability, small pinpoint white dots, single hairs or group of two hairs surrounded by a peripilar gray-white halo, and pigmented asterisk-like macules with sparse terminal and vellus-like hairs. Absence of follicular openings is not immediately evident because of the presence of pinpoint white dots. Careful examination, however, shows that the pinpoint white dots have an irregular distribution in addition to irregular white patches where the dots are absent. The alopecic area is not completely devoid of hair, but shows vellus and miniaturized and some terminal hairs. These often emerge grouped in twos and surrounded by a white-gray halo (**Fig. 6**).[10,22]

TRACTION ALOPECIA

Persistent hair traction is a common problem affecting African American women and children due to hair grooming practices and hairstyle preferences that result in increased tension on the hair.[23,24] This traction often leads to the formation of hair casts (**Fig. 7**). These casts are small, mobile, cylindrical structures enveloping the proximal hair shaft and may be mistaken for nits.[25,26] They appear white to brown in color and have spindled edges.[27] Their presence at the periphery of the alopecic patch indicates ongoing traction and suggests that the alopecia is likely to progress.[27] Making the diagnosis of marginal alopecia in African American women is relatively straightforward. Dermoscopy, however, can confirm that the cause of traction has not been removed and it can help convince the patient of the necessity to change hairstyle. Furthermore, hair casts are difficult to distinguish from scalp scaling without dermatoscopy.[27]

Dermoscopy of the alopecic area shows reduced hair density with numerous miniaturized hairs and pinpoint white dots.[27]

DISCOID LUPUS ERYTHEMATOSUS

In discoid lupus erythematosus (DLE), early and accurate diagnosis is critical because untreated

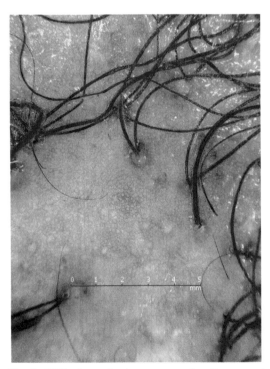

Fig. 6. CCCA: the scalp shows areas of erythema and pinpoint white dots with irregular distribution. The alopecic area shows single hairs or group of two hairs surrounded by a peripilar gray-white halo.

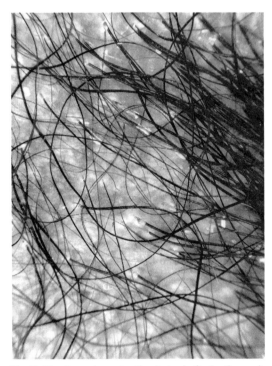

Fig. 7. Traction alopecia: the hair shafts in the scalp that surround the alopecic area show hair casts around their proximal part.

disease can often lead to significant scarring and atrophy. On trichoscopy, the affected areas show a reduction in the number of pinpoint white dots with evident scarring. This is secondary to significant involvement of the sweat glands in DLE compared with LPP in which sweat ducts are not involved. Follicular keratotic plugs are another typical dermoscopic finding of DLE.[28] Histopathologically, these areas with prominent follicular plugging correlate with hyperkeratosis as well as significant keratotic plugging of the follicular ostia at the level of the infundibulum. Importantly, these keratotic plugs may be found in areas of active or chronic alopecia; however, their presence can ultimately assist in differentiating scalp DLE from other scarring alopecias.[28] Also typical with DLE are blue-gray dots in a speckled pattern caused by involvement of the hair follicle and the interfollicular epidermis.[29]

LPP

In LPP, dermoscopy shows features similar to those described in CCCA; however, peripilar casts are typically observed around the terminal hairs within and surrounding the alopecic patches. The alopecia areas shows pinpoint white dots and white patches that correspond to follicular scars. Perifollicular blue-gray dots form an annular or target pattern.[29] On histology, the blue-gray dots demonstrate loose melanin or fine melanin particles within melanophages or free in the papillary dermis. The target pattern results from the accumulation of melanophages around the hair follicles, sparing the interfollicular epidermis.[29]

FRONTAL FIBROSING ALOPECIA

Frontal fibrosing alopecia (FFA) is a clinical variant of LPP, which typically affects postmenopausal women causing progressive recession of the frontotemporal hairline and loss of the eyebrows. In African descent women, it is often associated with traction alopecia.[30]

Dermoscopy is useful for fast diagnosis. In FFA, vellus hairs are typically absent at the hairline, which are characteristically preserved in traction alopecia. The terminal hairs at the new hairline demonstrate peripilar casts (**Fig. 8**). Black dots and broken hairs can also be seen.[31] The alopecic scalp shows the pinpoint white dots and white patches.

DISSECTING CELLULITIS OF THE SCALP

Dissecting cellulitis of the scalp (DCS) is a relapsing disease characterized by follicular occlusion.

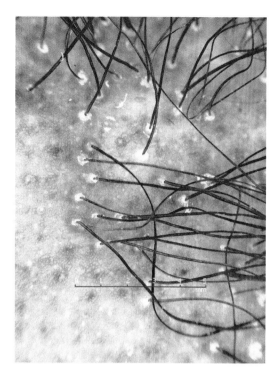

Fig. 8. FFA: peripilar casts and absence of vellus hairs.

Painful nodules and boggy plaques are characteristic of the disease. Initially, these lesions may be reversible; however, over time they result in scarring alopecia.[32] The disease most commonly affects black men in their third to fifth decades of life.[19] Dermatoscopy shows a pattern of nonscarring alopecia with regularly distributed pinpoint white dots, enlarged plugged follicular openings, and cadaverized hairs. It has been suggested that early DCS is characterized by anagen hair loss and that it demonstrates trichoscopic features similar to alopecia areata.[33] Histologically, there is a decrease in the number of anagen phase hair follicles with an increase in catagen or telogen follicles. Because of the increased premature transition to catagen stage, pigment casts can be found. At the level of the isthmus, there is a striking perifollicular inflammatory infiltrate, composed of lymphocytes, neutrophils, histiocytes, and plasma cells. Tosti and colleagues[33] suggest that this acute inflammation interrupts the rapidly dividing cells in their anagen phase, causing them to prematurely enter into telogen.

PILI ANNULATI

Pili annulati (PA) is a rare hair shaft abnormality, with fewer than 50 reported cases.[34] The hairs in PA appear shiny and speckled, with alternating light and dark bands under transmitted light microscopy.[35] Hair strength is usually unaffected and within normal limits; however, some patients experience increased vulnerability to weathering in the light band areas.[36] Although only a single case of PA has been reported in an African American patient, Osorio and colleagues[35] suggests that dermatoscopy may be useful in the diagnosis of this condition in patients with Afro-textured hair. They describe the aforementioned alternating light and dark bands on trichoscopy in a 49-year-old African American woman with PA. *T nodosa*, a sign of hair weathering, was also observed in this patient using dermatoscopy.[35]

WHEN TO BIOPSY

The use of trichoscopy has considerably decreased the need for biopsies in nonscarring alopecias. In particular, dermoscopy is useful in the differential diagnosis of patchy alopecia and allows to recognize alopecia areata even when the patches are very small or the hair shedding involves the entire scalp without evident patches. Dermoscopy is useful to differentiate early FFA, characterized by the absence of vellus hairs and presence of peripilar casts from traction alopecia in which vellus hairs are typically preserved.

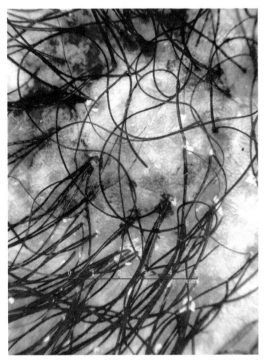

Fig. 9. Dermoscopy-guided biopsy in a patient with clinical suspicion of LPP. The biopsy site includes hairs with peripilar casts.

Biopsy is a critical step in the definitive diagnosis of all scarring alopecias. Dermoscopy is useful in selecting the biopsy site and ultimately increasing the rate of pathologic diagnosis. Dermoscopic features directing biopsy depend on clinical diagnosis and include one or two hairs emerging together, surrounded by a gray halo in CCCA, hair with peripilar casts in LPP (**Fig. 9**) and FFA, and keratotic plugs in DLE.[22] The dermoscopy-guided biopsy is particularly useful in women of African ancestry because they are often affected by more than one hair disorder. There is a high prevalence of certain conditions such as traction alopecia and CCCA in this population. The authors have many patients who had CCCA or traction alopecia for many years and then developed new patchy hair loss due to alopecia areata, TC, or even FFA. Dermoscopy helped in selecting the correct biopsy site for a definitive pathologic diagnosis.

SUMMARY

This article reviews the literature and provides extensive personal data on the usefulness of dermatoscopy in the systematic assessment of Afro-textured hair disorders. Increasing evidence supports trichoscopic evaluation in this population, particularly in cases that are otherwise clinically difficult to diagnose. This rapid, noninvasive technique can ultimately lead to earlier and more accurate diagnosis of hair disorders, as well as provide a convenient mode of follow-up. Further investigation is needed to enhance understanding of scalp disease in patients with Afro-textured hair.

REFERENCES

1. Ross EK, Vincenzi C, Tosti A. Videodermoscopy in the evaluation of hair and scalp disorders. J Am Acad Dermatol 2006;55(5):799–806.
2. Lacarrubba F, Dall'Oglio F, Rita Nasca M, et al. Videodermatoscopy enhances diagnostic capability in some forms of hair loss. Am J Clin Dermatol 2004; 5(3):205–8.
3. Syed A, Kuhajda A, Ayoub H, et al. African-American hair: its physical properties and differences relative to Caucasian hair. Cosmet Toil 1995;110: 39–48.
4. Lindelof B, Forslind B, Hedblad MA, et al. Human hair form. Morphology revealed by light and scanning electron microscopy and computer aided three-dimensional reconstruction. Arch Dermatol 1988;124(9):1359–63.
5. Franbourg A, Hallegot P, Baltenneck F, et al. Current research on ethnic hair. J Am Acad Dermatol 2003; 48(Suppl 6):S115–9.

6. Tosti A, Duque-Estrada B. Dermoscopy in hair disorders. J Egypt Women Dermatol Soc 2010;7(1):1–4.

7. Kossard S, Zagarella S. Spotted cicatricial alopecia in dark skin. A dermoscopic clue to fibrous tracts. Australas J Dermatol 1993;34(2):49–51.

8. Sperling LC. Hair density in African Americans. Arch Dermatol 1999;135(6):656–8.

9. Wallace MP, de Berker DA. Hair diagnoses and signs: the use of dermatoscopy. Clin Exp Dermatol 2010;35(1):41–6.

10. Miteva M, Tosti A. Hair and scalp dermatoscopy. J Am Acad Dermatol 2012;67(5):1040–8.

11. Abraham LS, Pineiro-Maceira J, Duque-Estrada B, et al. Pinpoint white dots in the scalp: dermoscopic and histopathologic correlation. J Am Acad Dermatol 2010;63(4):721–2.

12. Ardigo M, Torres F, Abraham LS, et al. Reflectance confocal microscopy can differentiate dermoscopic white dots of the scalp between sweat gland ducts or follicular infundibulum. Br J Dermatol 2011; 164(5):1122–4.

13. Hughes R, Chiaverini C, Bahadoran P, et al. Corkscrew hair: a new dermoscopic sign for diagnosis of tinea capitis in black children. Arch Dermatol 2011;147(3):355–6.

14. Vazquez-Lopez F, Palacios-Garcia L, Argenziano G. Dermoscopic corkscrew hairs dissolve after successful therapy of Trichophyton violaceum tinea capitis: a case report. Australas J Dermatol 2012; 53(2):118–9.

15. Slowinska M, Rudnicka L, Schwartz RA, et al. Comma hairs: a dermatoscopic marker for tinea capitis: a rapid diagnostic method. J Am Acad Dermatol 2008;59(Suppl 5):S77–9.

16. Okuda C, Ito M, Sato Y. Fungus invasion into human hair tissue in black dot ringworm: light and electron microscopic study. J Invest Dermatol 1988;90(5): 729–33.

17. de Moura LH, Duque-Estrada B, Abraham LS, et al. Dermoscopy findings of alopecia areata in an African-American patient. J Dermatol Case Rep 2008;2(4):52–4.

18. Osorio F, Tosti A. Hair weathering, Part 1: hair structure and pathogenesis. Cosmet Dermatol 2011;24: 533–8.

19. Rodney IJ, Onwudiwe OC, Callender VD, et al. Hair and scalp disorders in ethnic populations. J Drugs Dermatol 2013;12(4):420–7.

20. Halder RM, Grimes PE, McLaurin CI, et al. Incidence of common dermatoses in a predominantly black dermatologic practice. Cutis 1983;32(4):388, 90.

21. Alexis AF, Sergay AB, Taylor SC. Common dermatologic disorders in skin of color: a comparative practice survey. Cutis 2007;80(5):387–94.

22. Miteva M, Tosti A. Dermoscopy guided scalp biopsy in cicatricial alopecia. J Eur Acad Dermatol Venereol 2013;27(10):1299–303.

23. Mulinari-Brenner F, Bergfeld WF. Hair loss: an overview. Dermatol Nurs 2001;13(4):269–72, 277–8.

24. Khumalo NP, Jessop S, Gumedze F, et al. Determinants of marginal traction alopecia in African girls and women. J Am Acad Dermatol 2008;59(3):432–8.

25. Scott MJ Jr, Roenigk HH Jr. Hair casts: classification, staining characteristics, and differential diagnosis. J Am Acad Dermatol 1983;8(1):27–32.

26. Kohn SR. Hair casts or pseudonits. JAMA 1977; 238(19):2058–9.

27. Tosti A, Miteva M, Torres F, et al. Hair casts are a dermoscopic clue for the diagnosis of traction alopecia. Br J Dermatol 2010;163(6):1353–5.

28. Lanuti E, Miteva M, Romanelli P, et al. Trichoscopy and histopathology of follicular keratotic plugs in scalp discoid lupus erythematosus. Int J Trichology 2012;4(1):36–8.

29. Duque-Estrada B, Tamler C, Sodre CT, et al. Dermoscopy patterns of cicatricial alopecia resulting from discoid lupus erythematosus and lichen planopilaris. An Bras Dermatol 2010;85(2):179–83.

30. Dlova NC, Jordaan HF, Skenjane A, et al. Frontal fibrosing alopecia: a clinical review of 20 black patients from South Africa. Br J Dermatol 2013; 169(4):939–41.

31. Miteva M, Whiting D, Harries M, et al. Frontal fibrosing alopecia in black patients. Br J Dermatol 2012; 167(1):208–10.

32. Ross EK, Shapiro J. Primary cicatricial alopecia. In: Blume-Peytavi U, Tosti A, Whiting D, et al, editors. Hair growth and disorders. Lepzig (Germany): Springer; 2008. p. 211–6.

33. Tosti A, Torres F, Miteva M. Dermoscopy of early dissecting cellulitis of the scalp simulates alopecia areata. Actas Dermosifiliogr 2013;104(1):92–3.

34. Giehl KA, Rogers MA, Radivojkov M, et al. Pili annulati: refinement of the locus on chromosome 12q24.33 to a 2.9-Mb interval and candidate gene analysis. Br J Dermatol 2009;160(3):527–33.

35. Osorio F, Tosti A. Pili annulati—what about racial distribution? Dermatol Online J 2012;18(8):10.

36. Giehl KA, Ferguson DJ, Dawber RP, et al. Update on detection, morphology and fragility in pili annulati in three kindreds. J Eur Acad Dermatol Venereol 2004; 18(6):654–8.

Traction Alopecia
How to Translate Study Data for Public Education—Closing the KAP Gap?

Paradi Mirmirani, MD[a,b,c],
Nonhlanhla P. Khumalo, MBChB, FCDerm (SA), PhD[d,]*

KEYWORDS

- Traction alopecia • Alopecia • Public education • KAP gap • Hair loss • Hair grooming
- African hair

KEY POINTS

- Traction alopecia is common but preventable.
- The risk of traction alopecia increases with symptomatic traction-based hairstyles and is highest when tight hairstyles are done on chemically treated hair.
- A simple public education message for at-risk populations and hairdressers is to keep traction hairstyles for short periods (maximum of 2 weeks) and such hairstyles should be worn infrequently, be completely painless, and preferably done on natural hair.
- Teaching on "hair loss prevention" should ideally be an essential component of all hairdressing school curricula.

INTRODUCTION

Hair is an integral part of physical appearance, identity, and self-esteem. Hair care routines vary with factors such as age, gender, ethnicity, and religion. Hairstyles can lead to hair loss. Traction alopecia (TA) is hair loss due to ongoing or repetitive tension on the hair and is commonly seen in women of African descent who have tightly curly or spiral hair (**Fig. 1**). Although prevalent, TA is preventable and with appropriate education and public awareness, could potentially be eradicated. In many individuals, the problem may have its beginnings in childhood when the hair is styled tightly by adults to keep it "neat" for extended periods or to avoid tangling. Years of unrecognized or subclinical inflammation may

eventually lead to permanent follicular loss. TA is the only alopecia that is "biphasic" with early disease nonscarring and reversible, whereas chronic disease is scarring and permanent; this unique feature of TA is a call to action for prevention and early treatment.

Various studies have documented risk factors and hair care practices associated with TA. Can this study data be translated into education and public awareness efforts to prevent a problem that may have its beginnings in the preteen years? Such efforts may be most effective when representative groups of an at-risk population are surveyed about their knowledge, attitudes, and practices (KAP) regarding the particular health care issue. Tailoring and delivering public education messages to decrease the incidence of TA,

Disclosure: The authors have no conflicts of interest to disclose.
[a] Department of Dermatology, The Permanente Medical Group, Vallejo, CA, USA; [b] Department of Dermatology, University of California, San Francisco, CA, USA; [c] Department of Dermatology, Case Western Reserve University, Cleveland, OH, USA; [d] Division of Dermatology Ward G23, Groote Schuur Hospital Main Road Observatory and the University of Cape Town, Western Province 7925, South Africa
* Corresponding author.
E-mail address: n.khumalo@uct.ac.za

Dermatol Clin 32 (2014) 153–161
http://dx.doi.org/10.1016/j.det.2013.12.003
0733-8635/14/$ – see front matter © 2014 Elsevier Inc. All rights reserved.

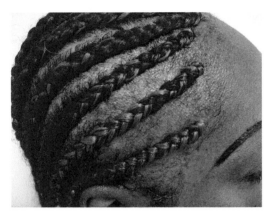

Fig. 1. Hair loss along the frontal marginal hairline due to prolonged use of hair braids.

and closing "the KAP gap" is a goal that is within reach and arguably more attainable in the age of Internet connectivity and social media.

CLINICAL PRESENTATION

Making the diagnosis of TA requires the clinician to have a high index of suspicion and to ask appropriate and clinically relevant questions of the patient and/or parents. In children, or in patients with early disease, there are often perifollicular papules and pustules in areas of the scalp with the highest tension (**Fig. 2**), but these lesions are often subclinical and go un-noticed.[1,2] However, if asked specifically, many patients will admit to having hairdressing symptoms, including tenderness, pimples, stinging, and crusting.[3,4] At the time of presentation, the patient may complain of sudden-onset patchy areas of hair loss and might deny any hair care practices that involve tension, which will often lead the clinician to a broad differential diagnosis. Clinical clues that should lead to further questions regarding hair care practices and TA include hair loss (most commonly noted along the marginal hairline: frontal, temporal, or occipital) with decreased but retained follicular markings and the presence of a "fringe" of finer, or miniaturized hairs (**Fig. 3**).[5] The presence of hair casts is a sign of ongoing or persistent TA.[1,6–8] Linear, curved, or geometric patterns of hair loss should also alert the clinician to the possibility of TA (**Fig. 4**).[2,9] TA may be unmasked by an episode of telogen effluvium; as a result, patients who may have had thinning hair in areas of traction but were able to style their hair in a cosmetically acceptable manner are no longer able to do so. In other instances, trauma to the hair, such as removal of a hair weave, can unmask TA[10]; presumably, follicles under tension are miniaturized,

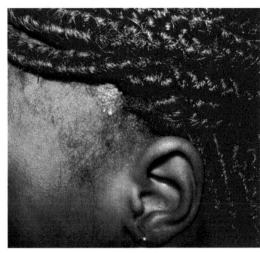

Fig. 2. Presence of perifollicular pustules in a child with early traction.

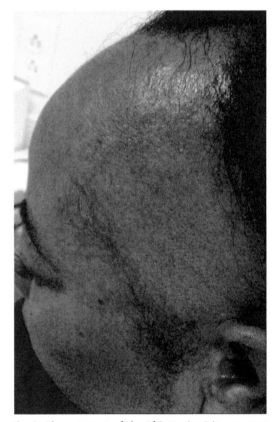

Fig. 3. The presence of the "fringe sign" in a woman with advanced traction alopecia. There is a margin of retained but finer, thinner-caliber hairs along the hairline and in front of the patch of alopecia. There are decreased but retained follicular markings in the area of alopecia.

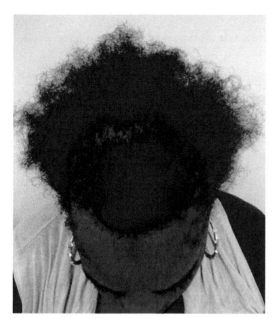

Fig. 4. A "horseshoe" or curved pattern of traction alopecia along the frontal scalp. The patient developed hair loss after placement of a weave.

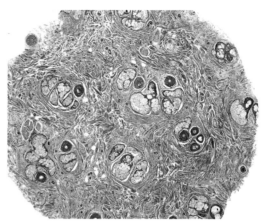

Fig. 5. Scalp biopsy from a patient with chronic traction alopecia showing reduced follicular density, follicular miniaturization, and retained sebaceous glands (hematoxylin-eosin, original magnification ×40). (*From* Samrao A, Price VH, Zedek D, et al. The "Fringe Sign"—A useful clinical finding in traction alopecia of the marginal hair line. Dermatol Online J 2011;17(11):1; with permission.)

or otherwise vulnerable and are unable to withstand additional stress.

HISTOLOGY

Because of the biphasic nature of TA, histologic changes in TA are variable and depend on the stage of disease. Reports of clinic-pathologic evaluations in TA are likely skewed toward late disease[11]; however, there is as yet no published data on the histopathologic spectrum of clinically graded mild to severe disease. In early TA, the histopathology shows trichomalacia, increased numbers of telogen and catagen hairs, a normal number of terminal follicles, and preserved sebaceous glands (Fig. 5).[5] Subsequently, there may be "follicular drop-out" of the terminal hairs where the follicles seem to have disappeared. The characteristic finding of retained but diminutive/smaller-caliber hairs along the frontal and/or temporal hairline (so-called fringe sign) may correlate with the vellus hairs seen on histology. With long-standing TA, sebaceous glands are present and vellus-sized hairs may be seen.[5,11,12] There is a decrease in the number of terminal follicles, which are replaced with fibrotic fibrous tracts. Inflammation is little to absent in long-standing TA, but may be mild in some cases of early TA. Transverse sections may offer advantages over vertical sections in distinguishing between primary scarring alopecias and TA.[13] Specifically, a diagnosis of TA should be considered if there is a low-power

pattern of miniaturization and follicular dropout with retained sebaceous glands.[14] In primary scarring, alopecias, the sebaceous glands, are absent in early-stage disease and even in clinically unaffected areas.[15]

DIFFERENTIAL DIAGNOSIS OF MARGINAL TRACTION ALOPECIA

TA may be misdiagnosed as ophiasis pattern alopecia areata (AA) or frontal fibrosing alopecia (FFA), because these disorders can have a similar bandlike pattern of hair loss along the marginal hairline.[5,10]

Clinical features that can help distinguish marginal TA from ophiasis pattern AA and FFA are summarized in Table 1. It should be emphasized that follicular markings or ostia are maintained in AA, often decreased in TA (especially late stage), and are absent in FFA (occasionally difficult to see). Eyebrows, body hair, skin, and nails are unaffected in TA, whereas they may be affected in both AA and FFA. As stated earlier, a biopsy is crucial in definitively distinguishing these entities.

DISEASE PREVALENCE

Recent studies have shed light on the high prevalence of disease. General population data has been reported from South Africa in cohorts of both children and adults.[3,4] In this population, mild to moderate TA is somewhat ubiquitous in females with up to one-third (31.7%) of adult women showing hair changes.[4] In children ages 6 to 15,

Table 1
A comparison of clinical features of traction alopecia, alopecia areata, and frontal fibrosing alopecia

	Traction Alopecia	Alopecia Areata	Frontal Fibrosing Alopecia
Follicular markings (ostia)	Decreased (especially in late-stage)	Retained	Absent/decreased
Perifollicular erythema	May be present in early stages	None	Typically present
Perifollicular scale	Scale or casts may be present in early or ongoing traction	None	Can be present
Hair findings	Fringe sign	Exclamation point hairs	Lonely hair sign[16]
Dermoscopy	Vellus hairs, mobile hair casts, pinpoint white dots	White pinpoint dots, yellow dots rarer in pigmented skin; exclamation mark hairs and black dots	Absence of vellus hairs, black dots and peripilar casts at new hairline
Appearance of scalp skin	Unchanged	May be slightly erythematous	Atrophic, sclerotic with accentuation of veins
Eyebrows	Unaffected	May be affected	Often affected
Body hair	Unaffected	May be affected	May be affected
Nail findings	None	Pits	None, pterygium (rare)
Skin findings	None	None	Lichen planus/lichen planus pigmentosus, facial papules, prominent facial veins
Mucosal findings	None	None	Oral lichen planus/ Wickham striae may be present

prevalence of disease ranges from 8.6% to 21.7%.[3] In a clinic population of African American girls aged 5.4 to 14.3 years, 18% showed signs of TA.[17]

CLINICAL TOOLS FOR QUANTIFYING DISEASE SEVERITY

The Marginal Traction Alopecia Severity Score (M-TAS) is a validated photographic scale developed to determine severity of marginal TA.[18] Both anterior and posterior hairlines are identified using anatomic landmarks and are graded on a scale of 0 to 9. The instrument has been used in clinical studies to correlate disease severity with potential risk factors for TA.[19] Potentially, the M-TAS can be a useful tool used to monitor response to treatment.

RISK FACTORS FOR TA
Hair Care Practices

An awareness and knowledge of hair care practices that can lead to TA is paramount in addressing this problem. **Table 2** lists common hair care practices that may lead to tension on the hair.[2,9,17,19–28] Unfortunately "excessive" tension is difficult to quantify, as each individual will have a different threshold at which there may be damage to the hair follicle. "Tenting," which occurs when the hair is pulled so tightly that the skin of the scalp is raised by the force of the pull, is a clear indication that there is excessive tension on the scalp and should be avoided.[5] Studies do suggest that the duration, length, and weight of hair or hair extensions may contribute to TA, as may the duration of wearing a certain hair style.[19] Sculpted hairstyles requiring multiple pins to keep the hair in place may also lead to traumatic hair loss,[29] as may use of pins used to fasten caps to the scalp (nurse's caps).[30,31]

In addition to hairstyles that cause tension, the hair may be subjected to chemicals and or heat in an effort to achieve a desired hairstyle.[32–34] Popular methods for straightening curly African hair include pressing or chemical relaxing (permanent).[3,4,32,33] Chemical relaxing/straightening products cleave the strong disulfide bonds using

Table 2
Common hair care practices that involve tension

Ponytails/pigtails	Hair or sections of hair pulled together and tied with an elastic band
Chignon	Hair pulled back and twisted, held with an elastic band or with pins
Braids	Small or large sections of hair that are interwoven. Extensions may or may not be added to braids
Cornrows	A style of braiding in which the hair sits close to the scalp
Twists	Sections of hair twisted onto itself and again twisted with another section
Sisterlocks	Sections of hair intertwined (using a tool similar to a crochet hook)
Dreadlocks	Sections of hair matted together
Weaves	Artificial or natural wefts (strip of hair sewn together like a curtain with a seam at the top) are sewn, glued, or clipped or otherwise attached to the hair
Extensions	Small strips of natural or artificial hair that are glued, braided, clipped, or otherwise attached to the hair
Curlers	Sections of hair wrapped around a cylindrical object for the purposes of styling the hair

an alkaline reducing agent and lead to weakening of the hair shaft.[33,34] Amino acid analysis of relaxed hair has shown a reduced cysteine content similar to that seen in the genetically fragile hair of trichothiodystrophy.[35,36]

Heat may be applied indirectly to the hair (blow dryer, hood hair dryer) or directly (curling iron, hot comb, flat iron, hot curlers). Implements that apply heat directly to the hair are especially damaging and can lead to hair shaft disorders and hair breakage.[37,38] Another common chemical process that is frequently used is the application of hair dye. Permanent hair dye can cause damage to the hair due to the oxidation reaction that occurs in the hair shaft.[39] It is not recommended to have 2 different chemical processes done at the same time (ie, avoid dye and relaxer at the same time). Likewise, the application of heat to chemically processed hair can lead to destruction of the hair shaft.

Study data clearly show that TA is increased in those who have hair care practices that include tension or that combine chemicals or heat along with tension.[3,4,17,19] Among school girls in South Africa, rates of TA are higher in those with relaxed versus natural hair (22% vs 5.2%).[3] TA risk in African girls and women is highest for combined hairstyles (ie, traction [braids/weaves/locks] done on relaxed hair, odds ratio [OR] 3.47, $P<.001$, confidence interval [CI] 1.94–6.20).[19] Among African American girls, TA risk was also significantly increased with traction and a history of relaxers (OR 5.27, CI 1.5–18.32, $P = .009$).[17]

The frequency of shampooing, use of pomades or hair products has not been shown to be associated with an increased risk of TA.[17] However, baseline scalp sebum in both women with Afro-textured and natural hair is a proinflammatory state: interleukin-1alpha (IL-1α) is 18 times higher than IL-1 receptor antagonist (IL-1ra).[40] The proinflammatory state maybe related to the moisturizers, although this needs validation.

Hair Type

Although TA occurs more commonly in women of African descent who have tight curly (spiral) black hair, studies suggest that increased risk of disease is associated with hair care practices, as opposed to hair types. Hair types are commonly divided into 3 categories: "black/African," Caucasian, Asian. The term "Afro-textured" is also used to refer to black or African hair that is tightly curled. Other classifications have been suggested based on the shape or degree of curl of the hair instead of race.[41,42] There are no significant biochemical differences among the hair types, with each showing a similar amino acid content and homogeneity of the structural organization of hair keratin; however, a number of other morphologic and histologic differences have been noted.[43–47] African hair has different hair growth parameters compared with Caucasian hair, specifically decreased density and hair growth rates and increased telogen hairs.[48] A comparison of scalp biopsies from Caucasian and African American patients without clinical hair loss showed a decreased overall hair density and fewer terminal follicles.[49] Follicles in African hair are curved compared with straight follicles in Caucasians and produce elliptical instead of oval hair shafts.[50] African hair has a high degree of variability in diameter compared with Asian and Caucasian hair, which impacts the mechanical properties.[47] The flattened elliptical shape of the hair shaft is likely responsible for the observation that the tensile strength of African hair is decreased compared with straight hair.[47] Additionally, African hair shows a greater tendency to form knots and fissures compared with Caucasian and Asian hair.[51]

Further supporting the concept that it is hair care that leads to TA and not hair type is the fact that TA has been reported in people of different races and ethnicities with different hair types. TA has been described in patients from Greenland who developed hair loss along the hairline because of the prolonged wearing of tight ponytails.[21] A similar pattern has been described in Hispanic women.[5] Frontal and parietal alopecia has been described in Sikh males as a result of twisting their uncut hair tightly on the scalp; submandibular TA has also been reported in a Sikh male who tied his beard in a tight knot below the chin.[40,52,53] TA confined to the occipital or temporal scalp due to "chignon" buns has been described in European women.[27,28] TA in Amish American women is noted on the temporal scalp where the religious head dressing is pinned (Paradi Mirmirani, personal observation, 2013).

Genetic Factors

It has been suggested that TA occurs more commonly in patients with a family history of androgenetic alopecia (AGA).[27] Indeed, vellus-sized or miniaturized follicles are typically noted on scalp biopsy along with follicular dropout.[5,12,14] Whether these miniaturized follicles represent androgen-mediated changes or whether pathologic mechanisms associated with TA can lead to miniaturization is not clear, but the evidence seems to support the latter. Although miniaturization is seen in both conditions, follicular miniaturization is more prominent and the number of terminal follicles is greater in AGA than in long-standing TA. In one series of patients with TA, only 5% were noted to have concomitant AGA on clinical examination.[5] Considering the known plasticity of the hair follicle and the fact that the size of the hair follicle changes over time and is determined by the size of the dermal papilla, it is conceivable that chronic traction may affect the dermal papilla and lead to a diminution of the hair follicle.

Hairdressing Symptoms

The risk of TA increases with symptomatic traction. When asked about symptoms starting during hairdressing, only 18.9% of patients with TA

denied having either tight painful braids, tight painful braids resulting in pimples, stinging from relaxer, or stinging from relaxer resulting in crusts.[19] The risk of TA increases with symptomatic traction (pain, pimples, crusts) (OR 1.98, P<.022, CI 1.10–3.57).[19]

Age

TA has been reported to occur in a child as young as 8 months of age.[2] Although TA is seen in school-aged children, the prevalence increases with age and is highest among adult women (Fig. 6).

Gender

The prevalence is higher in African schoolgirls than boys (17.1% vs 0%),[3] and is higher in women as compared with men (31.7% in women vs 2.3% in men; with affected men more likely to wear cornrows and dreadlocks).[4]

TREATMENT OPTIONS

Treatment options for TA vary depending on whether or not long-standing disease has resulted in permanent hair loss. Treatment can be divided into 3 stages: prevention, early TA, and long-standing TA.[5] Prevention strategies and educational messages should be aimed at parents of children and adolescents, as well as young adults, as these are years during which hair follicles may be most vulnerable and hair care practices, attitudes, and practices are forming.

In children and adults with early TA where the follicular unit is presumably still intact, it is important to loosen the hairstyle, and avoid chemicals

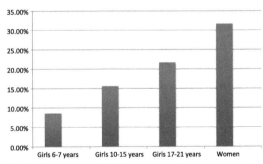

Fig. 6. Frequency of TA in a population of school children and adults 8.6% (6–7 years), 15.6% (10–15 years), to 21.7% (17–21 years) adult women (31.7%). (*Data from* Khumalo NP, Jessop S, Gumedze F, et al. Hairdressing is associated with scalp disease in African schoolchildren. Br J Dermatol 2007;157(1):106–10; and Khumalo NP, Jessop S, Gumedze F, et al. Hairdressing and the prevalence of scalp disease in African adults. Br J Dermatol 2007;157(5):981–8.)

or heat because cessation of tension can lead to hair regrowth. Brushing the affected area "to stimulate hair growth" should be avoided. There is little evidence-based data for pharmacologic treatment of TA. Use of topical or intralesional corticosteroids are recommended if there is any evidence of inflammation, such as scaling or erythema or symptoms of scalp tenderness.[5,22,54] Intralesional triamcinolone is directed at the periphery of hair loss.[54] Oral or topical antibiotics also may be used in the early stages of disease for their anti-inflammatory effect, especially if there is clinical evidence of pustules.[54] Case reports have shown a promising role for 2% topical minoxidil in the promotion of hair growth in patients with TA.[55] In our practice (P.M.) we frequently recommend a trial of minoxidil 5% applied carefully once daily to avoid hypertrichosis of the forehead.

In long-standing disease, surgical options may be considered. Hair transplants, in the form of micro-grafting, mini-grafting, and follicular unit transplantation, have been effective.[25,54,56] The surgical treatment of hair loss is discussed in detail elsewhere in this issue.

PUBLIC EDUCATION STRATEGIES

Education strategies and health care policies aimed at improving public health have often relied on identifying current knowledge, attitudes, and practices (KAP) in the population of concern. By surveying KAP, the efficacy of subsequent public education efforts or other interventions can be measured and quantified. Multiple situations have been identified in which health issues persist despite extensive medical knowledge. Common examples include the prevalence of smoking despite knowledge of health hazards, the poor control of diabetes despite the detrimental effects of hyperglycemia, and risky sexual behaviors despite knowledge of human immune deficiency virus transmission. In these cases, although theoretical knowledge of the health care issues exist, the attitude of patients and health care providers may influence changes in behavior or practices. Thus, the strategy of public health efforts has focused on closing the "KAP gap."

Although there has been extensive research on potential risk factors for TA, there is still a high prevalence of disease, indicating that there may be a "KAP gap" that could be bridged with educational campaigns. The largest "at-risk" population for TA includes children, adolescents, and young adults with Afro-textured hair. However, other targets for educational efforts could include parents of young children and hairdressers. One study surveyed the interest of hairdressers in participating in skin cancer education programs and found them to be receptive partners.[57] A recent South African survey identified 14 hairdressing schools in the greater Cape Town area. Of the 10 schools that responded to the survey, 7 taught African hair and 3 list "scalp disease" as a tutorial but none had a section on hair loss prevention (Nonhlanhla P. Khumalo, unpublished data, 2013).

Table 3
Doctor's orders to prevent Traction Alopecia and the "Fringe Sign"

Contributor	Best Option	Compromise
Traction Hairstyle symptoms (pain, tenderness, discomfort)	Tell hairdresser to loosen immediately, undo if pain noticed later	None No damp scarves, aspirin or paracetamol
Relaxers	Avoid completely, especially in children (hair damage increases with exposure duration)	Apply according to package instructions; process only the new growth or "virgin hair," no "smoothing" of the cream through previously relaxed hair. Thoroughly rinse and neutralize after processing or immediately if scalp tingling or burning occurs.
	No traction hairstyles (relaxed hair is weak, breaks easily)	>2 wk after processing, no pain
Hair dyes	On natural hair Avoid completely on relaxed hair (compounds damage)	On relaxed hair >2 wk after processing
Heat	Avoid especially hot combs and flat irons on relaxed/dyed hair–air dry	Low heat settings, infrequently

Although more research is required, currently known risk factors for TA could be translated for clear preventive public health messages (Table 3).[58]

SUMMARY

Some potential avenues for disseminating public health messages about prevention of TA could include use of the media, social media, and educational partnerships between hairdressing and health care organizations. However, there is an urgent need to lobby for dedicated teaching on hair loss prevention to be made an essential component of all hairdressing school curricula.

REFERENCES

1. Rollins TG. Traction follicultis with hair casts and alopecia. Am J Dis Child 1961;101:639–40.
2. Fox GN, Stausmire JM, Mehregan DR. Traction folliculitis: an underreported entity. Cutis 2007; 79(1):26–30.
3. Khumalo NP, Jessop S, Gumedze F, et al. Hairdressing is associated with scalp disease in African schoolchildren. Br J Dermatol 2007;157(1): 106–10.
4. Khumalo NP, Jessop S, Gumedze F, et al. Hairdressing and the prevalence of scalp disease in African adults. Br J Dermatol 2007;157(5):981–8.
5. Samrao A, Price VH, Zedek D, et al. The "Fringe Sign"—A useful clinical finding in traction alopecia of the marginal hair line. Dermatol Online J 2011; 17(11):1.
6. Tosti A, Miteva M, Torres F, et al. Hair casts are a dermoscopic clue for the diagnosis of traction alopecia. Br J Dermatol 2010;163(6):1353–5.
7. Ozuguz P, Kacar S, Takci Z, et al. Generalized hair casts due to traction. Pediatr Dermatol 2013;30(5): 614–5.
8. Zhang W. Epidemiological and aetiological studies on hair casts. Clin Exp Dermatol 1995;20(3):202–7.
9. Ahdout J, Mirmirani P. Weft hair extensions causing a distinctive horseshoe pattern of traction alopecia. J Am Acad Dermatol 2012;67(6):e294–5.
10. Heath CR, Taylor SC. Alopecia in an ophiasis pattern: traction alopecia versus alopecia areata. Cutis 2012;89(5):213–6.
11. Goldberg LJ. Cicatricial marginal alopecia: is it all traction? Br J Dermatol 2009;160(1):62–8.
12. Sperling LC, Lupton GP. Histopathology of non-scarring alopecia. J Cutan Pathol 1995;22(2): 97–114.
13. Donovan JC, Mirmirani P. Transversely sectioned biopsies in the diagnosis of end-stage traction alopecia. Dermatol Online J 2013;19(4):11.
14. Miteva M, Tosti A. 'A detective look' at hair biopsies from African-American patients. Br J Dermatol 2012;166(6):1289–94.
15. Mirmirani P, Willey A, Headington JT, et al. Primary cicatricial alopecia: histopathologic findings do not distinguish clinical variants. J Am Acad Dermatol 2005;52(4):637–43.
16. Tosti A, Miteva M, Torres F. Lonely hair: a clue to the diagnosis of frontal fibrosing alopecia. Arch Dermatol 2011;147(10):1240.
17. Rucker Wright D, Gathers R, Kapke A, et al. Hair care practices and their association with scalp and hair disorders in African American girls. J Am Acad Dermatol 2011;64(2):253–62.
18. Khumalo NP, Ngwanya RM, Jessop S, et al. Marginal traction alopecia severity score: development and test of reliability. J Cosmet Dermatol 2007;6(4): 262–9.
19. Khumalo NP, Jessop S, Gumedze F, et al. Determinants of marginal traction alopecia in African girls and women. J Am Acad Dermatol 2008;59(3): 432–8.
20. Lipnik MJ. Traumatic alopecia from brush rollers. Arch Dermatol 1961;84:493–5.
21. Hjorth N. Traumatic marginal alopecia; a special type: alopecia groenlandica. Br J Dermatol 1957; 69(9):319–22.
22. Fu JM, Price VH. Approach to hair loss in women of color. Semin Cutan Med Surg 2009;28(2):109–14.
23. Hantash BM, Schwartz RA. Traction alopecia in children. Cutis 2003;71(1):18–20.
24. Harman RR. Traction alopecia due to "hair extension". Br J Dermatol 1972;87(1):79–80.
25. Ozcelik D. Extensive traction alopecia attributable to ponytail hairstyle and its treatment with hair transplantation. Aesthetic Plast Surg 2005;29(4): 325–7.
26. Yang A, Iorizzo M, Vincenzi C, et al. Hair extensions: a concerning cause of hair disorders. Br J Dermatol 2009;160(1):207–9.
27. Trueb RM. "Chignon alopecia": a distinctive type of nonmarginal traction alopecia. Cutis 1995;55(3):178–9.
28. Samrao A, Chen C, Zedek D, et al. Traction alopecia in a ballerina: clinicopathologic features. Arch Dermatol 2010;146(8):930–1.
29. Ntuen E, Stein SL. Hairpin-induced alopecia: case reports and a review of the literature. Cutis 2010; 85(5):242–5.
30. Hwang SM, Lee WS, Choi EH, et al. Nurse's cap alopecia. Int J Dermatol 1999;38(3):187–91.
31. Renna FS, Freedberg IM. Traction alopecia in nurses. Arch Dermatol 1973;108(5):694–5.
32. McMichael AJ. Ethnic hair update: past and present. J Am Acad Dermatol 2003;48(Suppl 6):S127–33.
33. Quinn CR, Quinn TM, Kelly AP. Hair care practices in African American women. Cutis 2003;72(4):280–2, 285–9.

34. Bolduc C, Shapiro J. Hair care products: waving, straightening, conditioning, and coloring. Clin Dermatol 2001;19(4):431–6.

35. Khumalo NP, Stone J, Gumedze F, et al. 'Relaxers' damage hair: evidence from amino acid analysis. J Am Acad Dermatol 2010;62(3):402–8.

36. Beach RA, Wilkinson KA, Gumedze F, et al. Sebum transforming growth factor beta1 induced by hair products. Arch Dermatol 2012;148(6):764–6.

37. Mirmirani P. Ceramic flat irons: improper use leading to acquired trichorrhexis nodosa. J Am Acad Dermatol 2010;62(1):145–7.

38. Ruetsch SB, Kamath YK. Effects of thermal treatments with a curling iron on hair fiber. J Cosmet Sci 2004;55(1):13–27.

39. Draelos ZK. Hair cosmetics. Dermatol Clin 1991; 9(1):19–27.

40. Beach RA, Wilkinson KA, Gumedze F, et al. Baseline sebum IL-1alpha is higher than expected in afro-textured hair: a risk factor for hair loss? J Cosmet Dermatol 2012;11(1):9–16.

41. Loussouarn G, Garcel AL, Lozano I, et al. Worldwide diversity of hair curliness: a new method of assessment. Int J Dermatol 2007;46(Suppl 1):2–6.

42. De la Mettrie R, Saint-Leger D, Loussouarn G, et al. Shape variability and classification of human hair: a worldwide approach. Hum Biol 2007;79(3): 265–81.

43. Lindelof B, Forslind B, Hedblad MA, et al. Human hair form. Morphology revealed by light and scanning electron microscopy and computer aided three-dimensional reconstruction. Arch Dermatol 1988;124(9):1359–63.

44. Dekio S, Jidoi J. Amounts of fibrous proteins and matrix substances in hairs of different races. J Dermatol 1990;17(1):62–4.

45. Khumalo NP. African hair morphology: macrostructure to ultrastructure. Int J Dermatol 2005; 44(Suppl 1):10–2.

46. Khumalo NP, Dawber RP, Ferguson DJ. Apparent fragility of African hair is unrelated to the cystine-rich protein distribution: a cytochemical electron microscopic study. Exp Dermatol 2005;14(4):311–4.

47. Franbourg A, Hallegot P, Baltenneck F, et al. Current research on ethnic hair. J Am Acad Dermatol 2003;48(Suppl 6):S115–9.

48. Loussouarn G. African hair growth parameters. Br J Dermatol 2001;145(2):294–7.

49. Sperling LC. Hair density in African Americans. Arch Dermatol 1999;135(6):656–8.

50. Bernard BA. Hair shape of curly hair. J Am Acad Dermatol 2003;48(Suppl 6):S120–6.

51. Khumalo NP, Doe PT, Dawber RP, et al. What is normal black African hair? A light and scanning electron-microscopic study. J Am Acad Dermatol 2000;43(5 Pt 1):814–20.

52. Kanwar AJ, Kaur S, Basak P, et al. Traction alopecia in Sikh males. Arch Dermatol 1989;125(11):1587.

53. James J, Saladi RN, Fox JL. Traction alopecia in Sikh male patients. J Am Board Fam Med 2007; 20(5):497–8.

54. Callender VD, McMichael AJ, Cohen GF. Medical and surgical therapies for alopecias in black women. Dermatol Ther 2004;17(2):164–76.

55. Khumalo NP, Ngwanya RM. Traction alopecia: 2% topical minoxidil shows promise. Report of two cases. J Eur Acad Dermatol Venereol 2007;21(3): 433–4.

56. Earles RM. Surgical correction of traumatic alopecia marginalis or traction alopecia in black women. J Dermatol Surg Oncol 1986;12(1):78–82.

57. Bailey EE, Marghoob AA, Orengo IF, et al. Skin cancer knowledge, attitudes, and behaviors in the salon: a survey of working hair professionals in Houston, Texas. Arch Dermatol 2011;147(10): 1159–65.

58. Khumalo NP. The "fringe sign" for public education on traction alopecia. Dermatol Online J 2012;18(9):16.

Advances and Challenges in Hair Restoration of Curly Afrocentric Hair

Nicole E. Rogers, MD[a,b], Valerie D. Callender, MD[c,d],*

KEYWORDS

- Hair restoration • Hair transplantation • Follicular unit extraction (FUE)
- Follicular unit transplantation (FUT) • Ethnic hair • Central centrifugal cicatricial alopecia (CCCA)
- Traction alopecia

KEY POINTS

- Although the biochemical composition of hair is similar among racial and ethnic groups, the hair structure between them varies.
- Individuals with curly hair pose specific challenges and special considerations when a surgical option for alopecia is considered.
- Hair restoration in this population should be approached with knowledge on the clinical characteristics of curly hair, hair grooming techniques that may influence the management, unique indications for the procedure, surgical instrumentation used, and the complications that may arise.

INTRODUCTION

Hair transplantation offers a permanent and dramatic effect for patients with thinning hair. The technique was originally conceived in the early to mid-1900s by hair transplant pioneers Dr Shoji Okuda[1,2] of Japan and Dr Norman Orentreich[3–5] of the United States. Since then, the cosmetic results of hair transplantation have improved with the refinement of graft size from punches of 4 to 5 mm to single follicular unit grafts of 1 to 4 hairs. Dr Bobby Limmer,[6] in his landmark article, revolutionized the field with the application of stereoscopic magnification for the separation of follicular units. Since then, the field has continued to evolve with surgical procedures such as follicular unit extraction (FUE) and the use of robotic technology as an efficient method of graft harvesting.

Most hair transplant surgeries are performed on persons of white ancestry with male or female pattern hair loss. According to the 2013 International Society of Hair Restoration Surgery practice census results, more than 310,000 hair transplant surgeries were performed worldwide: 86.3% in men and 13.7% in women.[7] As the demographics of the United States and developing world change, more persons of Afrocentric background will present for surgical treatment of their hair loss. Early pioneers of hair restoration realized that differences exist that must be understood before proceeding with surgery in this population.[8,9] These differences relate to the structure of the hair follicle, the role of hair grooming techniques, and the need to consider other factors such as scarring or keloid formation. This chapter considers the most common causes of hair loss in patients of African descent and focuses on the differences in surgical technique.

[a] Department of Dermatology, Tulane University School of Medicine, New Orleans, LA, USA; [b] Hair Restoration of the South, Metairie, LA, USA; [c] Howard University College of Medicine, 520 West Street Northwest, Washington, DC 20059, USA; [d] Callender Dermatology & Cosmetic Center, 12200 Annapolis Road, Suite 315, Glenn Dale, MD 20769, USA
* Corresponding author. Callender Dermatology and Cosmetic Center, 12200 Annapolis Road, Suite 315, Glenn Dale, MD 20769.
E-mail address: drcallender@callenderskin.com

Dermatol Clin 32 (2014) 163–171
http://dx.doi.org/10.1016/j.det.2013.12.004
0733-8635/14/$ – see front matter © 2014 Elsevier Inc. All rights reserved.

CANDIDATE SELECTION

The most common type of hair loss in Caucasian women is female pattern hair loss, a form of non-scarring alopecia. However, in women of African descent, most patients with hair loss have either central centrifugal cicatricial alopecia (CCCA) or traction alopecia. CCCA is an idiopathic primary scarring form of hair loss and is thought by the authors to have a genetic component, because it frequently runs in families (**Fig. 1**). In addition, it can potentially be worsened by environmental factors such as the use of chemical relaxers or heat-related treatments.[10–14] For this reason, patients with CCCA should first undergo medical therapy to minimize and control any active inflammation before surgery. In addition, proper hair grooming techniques should be followed. **Fig. 2** shows the dermatoscopic appearance of hair follicles before and after treatment with oral doxycycline and topical clobetasol to suppress the inflammation. A decrease in perifollicular erythema can be seen. Most hair transplant surgeons recommend a minimum of 9 to 12 months of medical therapy before hair transplantation.

Nonscarring causes of hair loss in patients of African descent are traction alopecia (TA) and female pattern hair loss. TA generally occurs as a result of traumatic grooming practices.[10–14] Tight braids, ponytails, dreadlocks, tracts, and weaves can cause loss of follicles along the frontal hairline, sideburn area, and occiput (ophiasis pattern). There is usually little inflammation and an absence of scarring in these two forms of hair loss. TA represents a secondary form of hair loss, as opposed to the primary inflammatory process of CCCA (**Table 1**).

MAJOR CONSIDERATIONS/DIFFERENCES

Table 2 lists the major differences between Afrocentric and Caucasian hair. Besides the obvious

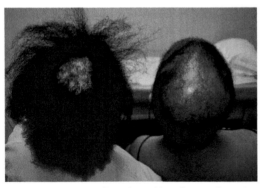

Fig. 1. Two sisters with early and late forms of scarring hair loss in the vertex area, shown on biopsy to be CCCA.

difference of curly hair in the African population, it has been observed that they have a smaller number of follicular units per square centimeter (lower density) and a slightly higher number of hairs per follicular unit. Because of these major differences, a larger recipient site must be created during hair transplant surgery. Also, more caution is needed in choosing surgical candidates given the higher risk of keloid formation in patients of African descent.

THE TEST TRANSPLANT

The authors have found the test transplant to be a valuable tool in identifying whether patients with scarring areas of hair loss may benefit from hair transplantation. Although it may seem counterintuitive, the use of larger punch grafts is not only cosmetically acceptable in patients of African descent (because of the curly nature of the surrounding hair) but seems to allow better survival of the transplanted grafts, especially in areas of scar tissue. It can also theoretically help to improve the quality of the recipient area by allowing the transfer of healthy stem cells found in sebaceous glands and adipose cells of the donor subcutaneous tissue.

Test transplanting may also be valuable for patients with a known history or strong family history of keloid formation. By harvesting a small group or number of grafts from the back and transplanting them to the affected areas of hair loss, the surgeon can make sure that the patient does not have any thick scar formation in either the donor or recipient areas. This technique should not be limited to patients of African descent; any person at risk of keloid formation may benefit from test transplantation.

The authors perform test transplantation by harvesting one or more 2-mm to 5-mm punch grafts of hair-bearing skin from the occipital scalp. After closing the defects with suture or staples, the punch grafts are then placed into recipient sites created with a slightly smaller (by 0.5–1 mm) punch trephines (**Fig. 3**) in areas of hair loss. If a biopsy has not already been done, the tissue removed from the recipient site can be sent to a pathologist to assess the degree of inflammation present. **Table 3** provides a guide for test punch graft donor and recipient size planning.

After the punch grafts have been removed, and depending on how well they stay in place, sutures may be needed to hold the larger grafts in place. Other doctors have used Steri-Strips with benzoin to hold the grafts in place. Smaller punch grafts generally stay securely in place and do not require sutures or Steri-Strips. Patients are then

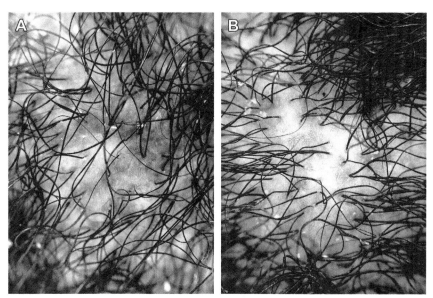

Fig. 2. Dermatoscopic exam: before (*A*) and after (*B*) medical therapy for CCCA.

encouraged to allow 3 to 6 months after the procedure to monitor for successful growth of the transplanted grafts. If the transplants are successful, the surgeon and patient may move forward with a larger hair transplant session, with more follicular units or punch grafts. Clinical photography is useful in documenting the response of the test procedure.

In areas where scarring is less of a concern, such as TA or female pattern hair loss, the smaller grafts containing single follicular units are more likely to be successful. Clinicians may harvest a single 8-mm punch from the back of the scalp and separate this punch graft into individual follicular units of 1 to 4 hairs. They can then be placed into 20 to 30 incisions 1.3 to 1.5 mm wide created in the recipient area (**Fig. 4**). Larger hair transplant sessions of hundreds of grafts can also be used in treating TA and female pattern hair loss. With either technique, patients are advised that it will likely take 6 to 12 months or more for the hairs to grow in.

Table 1 Common causes of hair loss in patients of African descent

Condition	Gender	Description	Location/Scale	Medical Therapy	Surgical Candidacy
Female pattern hair loss (AGA)	F	Nonscarring	Frontal one-third to two-thirds of the scalp; Ludwig I–III[15]	Topical minoxidil, OCPs, spironolactone, finasteride	Excellent
Male pattern hair loss (AGA)	M	Nonscarring	Bitemporal recession and vertex; Norwood I–VII[16]	Topical minoxidil, oral finasteride	Excellent
Traction alopecia	F>M	Nonscarring	Periauricular and bitemporal recession	Topical minoxidil, intralesional steroids	Usually good
CCCA	F>M	Inflammation and scarring	Vertex of scalp, expanding centrifugally	Doxycycline, topical steroids, intralesional steroids	Varies; test transplant recommended

Abbreviations: AGA, androgenetic alopecia; CCCA, central centrifugal cicatricial alopecia; F, female; M, male; OCPs, oral contraceptive pills.

Table 2 Differences between Afrocentric and Caucasian hair		
	Afrocentric Hair	Caucasian Hair
Follicle structure	Curved, coiled, helical or spiraled	Straight, wavy, or helical
Ratio of FU density	3	5[17]
Number of hairs per FU	3	2[18]
Recipient size	1.3–1.6 mm (2–4 mm for punch grafts)	0.8–1.3 mm
Incidence of keloids (%)	4.5–16[19]	0–3

Abbreviation: FU, follicular unit.

Table 3 Guide for test punch graft donor and recipient size planning	
Donor Punch Size (mm)	Recipient Punch Size (mm)
5	4 (disposable 4.5 punches do not exist)
4[a]	3.5
3	2.5
2	1.5

[a] Preferred method.

ANESTHESIA

Most patients do not need sedation and tolerate the procedure well under local anesthesia. Some patients may benefit from the addition of an anxiolytic such as diazepam but they cannot be allowed to drive after the procedure. In general, 1% to 2% lidocaine with 1:100,000 epinephrine is used to infiltrate the donor area before donor graft harvesting, which is first done along the most caudal aspect of the area to be harvested. The use of vibration can help alleviate pain via the gate theory. Then, long-acting bupivacaine is used along the periphery to minimize discomfort after removal of the donor grafts and throughout the rest of the procedure. Although bupivacaine has been known for cardiac toxicity, hair transplant surgery almost never requires as much as the 225-mg dose allowed with epinephrine 1:200,000 or the 175 mg allowed without epinephrine.[20]

For the recipient area, a 2% lidocaine ring block can help decrease the discomfort from subsequent injections. Also, the use of a triamcinolone suspension (3.3 mg of 10 mg/mL added to 1% lidocaine with epinephrine) can considerably reduce postoperative swelling in the forehead area.[21] The hair transplant surgeon should monitor total dosing to ensure that patients receive no more than 7.0 mg/kg body mass with epinephrine or 4.5 mg/kg body mass without epinephrine.[22] The authors recommend drawing up anesthetic in advance to control the amount used (**Fig. 5**).

DONOR HARVESTING

For patients who do not need a test transplant, or who have shown successful growth of

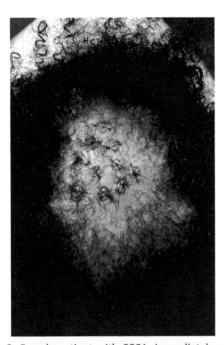

Fig. 3. Female patient with CCCA, immediately after placement of 10 test punch grafts.

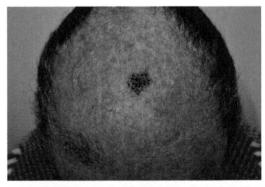

Fig. 4. Female patient with TA, after placement of 25 test follicular units of 1 to 4 hairs.

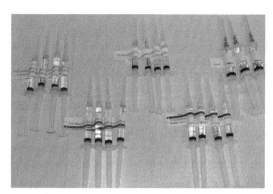

Fig. 5. Anesthetic drawn up and properly labeled in advance for hair transplantation.

test-transplanted hairs, the next step may be a standard elliptical excision from the hair-bearing occipital area. Immediately before the surgical excision, saline can be injected into the donor area to increase tissue turgor and make the tissue easier to separate. The authors do not recommend the use of a double-bladed scalpel for curly hair, because there is greater risk of transecting the donor follicles. Instead, a single 10 or 15 blade can be used to gently score the margins for harvest, going no more than 2 to 3 mm into the dermis. Then, the skin edges can be gently pulled apart using skin hooks in opposing angles. This technique of tension dissection allows the separation of the hair follicles located in the subcutaneous layer without the transection of follicles by a blade.

It is helpful to keep the width of the donor strip conservatively narrow (no wider than 1–1.5 cm) to help prevent an overly tight closure, which can result in wound dehiscence, tissue necrosis, or widened scar. In patients who have a history of smoking, diabetes, or poor wound healing, it is especially important to limit the tension on the donor wound. The resulting defect may be closed with dissolving suture, nylon suture, or staples. Removal of nylon suture or staples can occur as early as 7 to 10 days after surgery so long as there is evidence of good wound healing. Patients who undergo a conservative-width elliptical donor harvest can expect to heal with a fine, thin, horizontal scar in the donor area. This scar is usually of no cosmetic importance, and surrounding hair that is 1 to 2 cm long easily covers it.

GRAFT CREATION

After the donor ellipse has been harvested, a team of 1 to 4 or more technicians separates the strip into individual follicular units. This separation can be done with or without magnification, but excellent lighting and ergonomics are essential. The first step is to sliver the strip into narrow sections that are a single follicular unit wide (like slicing a loaf of bread). These narrow sections are then separated into 10 to 25 individual follicular units, depending on the density. Throughout the process the grafts should be kept moist and immersed in a saline solution. Even the slightest graft desiccation can have a major effect on graft survival.

As seen in **Fig. 6**, Afrocentric hair follicles typically have a C-shaped configuration within the skin. This configuration can make graft separation challenging and more time consuming, and specialized curved blades are helpful in separating the grafts. Rather than using straight 10 or 15 blades (on scalpel holders) or straight Personna blades (Personna Medical, Verona, VA) which are typically used for straight hair/follicles, it is helpful to either bend the Personna blades or use flexible Dermablades® (Personna Medical, Verona, VA) (**Fig. 7**).[23] This way the shape of the blade can be made to match the C-shaped curl of the hair follicle, as it occurs under the skin surface.

Most hair transplant surgeons use a simple saline solution to store the grafts in Petri dishes during the preparation process. Others chill the grafts, and still others use advanced holding solutions such as lactated ringer or HypoThermosol® (BioLife Solutions, Bothell, WA) containing various buffers, ATP, and glucose.[24] There are limited data showing the advantages of each of these solutions. However, it is well established that by minimizing the time out of the body, and by keeping the grafts well hydrated, 90% to 95% growth rate of transplanted follicles can be expected in nonscarred, noninflamed scalp.

HAIRLINE DESIGN

For men of color who seek surgical correction for their hair loss, the most commonly treated condition is androgenetic alopecia (AGA), or male

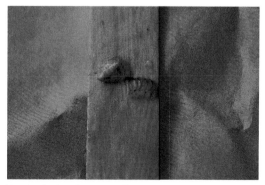

Fig. 6. Curly Afrocentric hair on a tongue blade from side view.

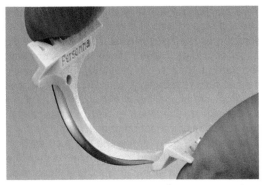

Fig. 7. The flexible DermaBlade® can be used to separate curly hair follicles. (*Courtesy of* Energizer Personal Care-Personna Medical, Verona, VA; with permission.)

pattern hair loss. This condition can present as hair thinning in a bitemporal distribution, recession of the frontal hairline, and/or hair thinning in the vertex area (**Fig. 8**). Because of the few cases of male hair loss involving inflammation or scarring[25] (ie, CCCA), hair transplantation can be done using individual follicular unit grafts rather than larger punch grafts. All patients are encouraged to allow for a masculine, age-appropriate hairline, which is not too low or too rounded in the temporal recessions. In general, men of color tend to prefer a more straight-across hairline. However, they must understand that, with age, the hairline may move back and require additional surgeries. Oral finasteride (1 mg) or topical 5% minoxidil may prevent or mitigate the ongoing hair loss.

Although some women of color present for hair transplant for female pattern hair loss, most present for surgical treatment of TA or CCCA. In TA, vestiges of the original hairline are frequently still evident by soft vellus or short broken hairs. These hairs can be used as an outline to fill in the areas of thinning with thicker, terminal hairs from the occipital scalp.

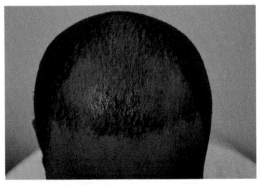

Fig. 8. Young African man with inherited hair loss (androgenetic alopecia).

For male or female patients with scarring or nonscarring hair loss in the vertex (crown), we recommend transplanting from the frontal area caudally. This way, as the hair grows in, it can at least be combed backward to help give improved coverage. Young men with AGA should be cautioned that loss of surrounding hair may result in an unnatural island of transplanted hair. Most surgeons do not transplant men with vertex thinning unless they are at least in their 50s, given the unpredictability of future hair loss and risk of a poor cosmetic outcome.

For women with CCCA, there is also less risk of graft failure when the hairs are transplanted predominantly in the central burned-out areas. Patients must understand that the periphery of CCCA-affected areas may flare up at any time. Thus, without concurrent medical treatment, the more peripherally placed follicles may grow initially, but then shed later, or fail to take. **Fig. 9** shows successful hair transplantation of an African woman with CCCA.

RECIPIENT SITE CREATION

While the surgical assistants are separating the grafts, the surgeon should be anesthetizing the recipient area of the scalp and creating small incisions in the scalp where the grafts will be inserted. Depending on the size and number of hairs per follicular unit, a slighter wider berth is generally needed for placement of curly hairs. The authors generally use steel blades or needles that vary in size from 1.2 to 1.5 mm. Simple 16-gauge to 18-gauge needles can work well, but may dull easily. Minde (1.3 or 1.5 mm wide) or spear-point blades (90 or 91) offer longer lasting, sharper cutting edges (**Fig. 10**).

GRAFT PLACEMENT

Specialized forceps are used to grasp the grafts gently just above the bulb, and then slide them into the recipient sites using a 2-handed technique with a Q-tip or gauze. Care should be taken not to pinch the bulb, twist the follicles, or bend them in half during placement. Even the slightest bit of desiccation can result in loss of graft viability. For this reason, grafts should remain immersed in a Petri dish solution until they are ready for placement. Some issues of graft popping may occur if patients have increased blood pressure, are on blood thinners, or if the recipient sites are too narrow or too shallow. Popping usually resolves by reinforcing the area with anesthetic containing epinephrine as well as gently holding pressure after graft placement. Care should be taken not

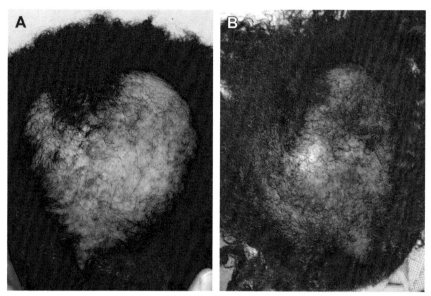

Fig. 9. (*A*) A 47-year-old African woman with CCCA before hair transplant surgery. (*B*) The same patient after undergoing hair transplantation with a total of 1124 follicular unit grafts of 1 to 4 hairs. This larger session was only performed after a test transplant showed successful growth.

to lodge the grafts too deeply (which can result in pitting) or not deeply enough (which can result in tenting). The top of the placed grafts should ideally sit approximately 1 mm above the surrounding skin.

POSTOPERATIVE CARE

Patients are advised to keep their heads slightly elevated the first night after surgery and to minimize vigorous exercise for 3 to 5 days after surgery. They may rinse the scalp with warm water for 3 days and start shampooing on the third day. A topical antibiotic ointment can be applied

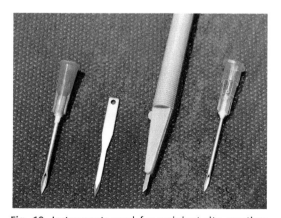

Fig. 10. Instruments used for recipient site creation. From left to right: 16-gauge needle (1.6 mm wide), spear-point blade 90 (1.5 mm wide), Minde knife (1.3 mm wide), 18-gauge needle (1.44 mm wide).

to the donor area to optimize wound healing of the donor scar. We explain that they will have some scabbing in the recipient area for 1 to 3 weeks after surgery. The duration of scabbing may be lessened by spraying with saline solution several times daily. Depending on the amount and location of anesthesia used, patients may have some forehead swelling. This swelling can be mitigated by including triamcinolone suspension with the anesthetic used.[21] Patients may also be instructed to ice the forehead, and/or be given a 3-day to 4-day course of oral or intramuscular corticosteroids to help prevent this swelling.

FUTURE TRENDS

Follicular unit extraction (FUE) is a new form of donor harvest used for patients who wear their hair short and do not want to have a linear scar at the donor site. It may also be used for patients with thin donor areas in which a scar would be obvious even with hair grown longer. It involves the use of 0.8-mm to 1-mm punch grafts to harvest single follicular units. The hairs are then placed in the recipient area as with a donor ellipse harvest. The procedure can be done manually but can be laborious. Several surgeries may be required to transplant the same number of follicles as with an elliptical donor harvest. This procedure should be used with caution in patients with curly hair because the size of the punch that is used for donor harvesting may cause transection of the hair follicle.[26]

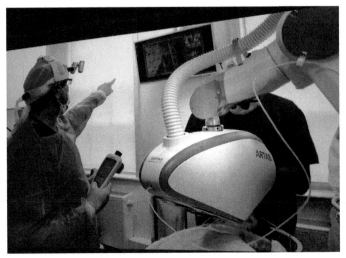

Fig. 11. Demonstration of the ARTAS robotic harvesting of hairs using automated technologies for rapid FUE. (*Courtesy of* R. Shapiro, MD and Restoration Robotics, Inc., San Jose, CA; with permission.)

Automated devices have emerged to make the FUE process more efficient. The ARTAS system uses sophisticated laser technology to calculate the angle of the emerging hair follicle, and a robot arm then punches out the graft (**Fig. 11**). A technician then carefully extracts the graft from the surrounding tissue. The use of this machine can result in the successful harvest of as many as 500 to 700 grafts per hour. The cost and space requirements of this device have so far limited its widespread implementation. Hair transplant surgeons must still understand and implement the fundamentals of hairline design and graft placement for optimal results.

So far, the FUE procedure (whether done manually or via automation) seems to have a limited use in treating patients with curly hair because the straight 0.8-mm to 1-mm punch grafts inevitably transect curly hairs. Even in Caucasian or Asian hair, transection rates ranging from 1.7% to 15% have been reported.[27] Although studies are lacking, the technique has presumably not been used much in the curly-hair population for this reason. Furthermore, it is not popular among women because it involves shaving a large donor area before harvesting.

SUMMARY

Although the biochemical composition of hair is similar among racial and ethnic groups, the hair structure between them varies, and individuals with curly hair pose specific challenges and special considerations when a surgical option for alopecia is considered. Hair restoration in this population should therefore be approached with knowledge on the clinical characteristics of curly hair, hair grooming techniques that may influence the management, unique indications for the procedure, surgical instrumentation used, and the complications that may arise.

REFERENCES

1. Okuda S. Clinical and experimental studies of transplantation of living hairs. Jpn J Dermatol Urol 1939; 46:1–11 [in Japanese].
2. Inui S, Itami S. Dr. Shoji Okuda (1886-1962): the great pioneer of punch graft hair transplantation. J Dermatol 2009;36:561–2.
3. Orentreich N. Autografts in alopecias and other selected dermatological conditions. Ann N Y Acad Sci 1959;83:463–79.
4. Orentreich N, Orentreich D. Androgenetic alopecia and its treatment-a historical overview. In: Unger WP, editor. Hair transplantation. 3rd edition. New York: Marcel Dekker Inc; 1995. p. 1–33.
5. Unger WP. The history of hair transplantation. Dermatol Surg 2000;26:181–9.
6. Limmer BL. Elliptical donor stereoscopically assisted micrografting as an approach to further refinement in hair transplantation. J Dermatol Surg Oncol 1994;20:789–93.
7. International Society of Hair Restoration Surgery 2013 Practice census facts and figures. Available at: http://www.ishrs.org/press-release/ishrs-2013-practice-census-facts-and-figures. Accessed September 30, 2013.
8. Selmanowitz VJ, Orentreich N. Hair transplantation in blacks. J Natl Med Assoc 1973;65:471–82.
9. Pierce HE. The uniqueness of hair transplantation in black patients. J Natl Med Assoc 1976;68:343.

10. Borovicka JH, Thomas L, Prince C, et al. Scarring alopecia: clinical and pathologic study of 54 African-American women. Int J Dermatol 2009;48:840–5.

11. Gathers RC, Lim HW. Central centrifugal cicatricial alopecia: past, present, and future. J Am Acad Dermatol 2008;60:660–8.

12. Callender VD, McMichael AJ, Cohen GF. Medical and surgical therapies for alopecias in black women. Dermatol Ther 2004;17:164–76.

13. Khumalo NP, Jessop S, Gumedze F, et al. Determinants of marginal traction alopecia in African girls and women. J Am Acad Dermatol 2008;59:432–8.

14. Khumalo NP, Jessop S, Gumedze F, et al. Hairdressing and the prevalence of scalp disease in African adults. Br J Dermatol 2007;157:981–8.

15. Ludwig E. Classification of the types of androgenetic alopecia. (common baldness) occurring in the female sex. Br J Dermatol 1977;97:247–54.

16. Norwood OT. Male pattern baldness: classification and incidence. South Med J 1975;68:1359–65.

17. Sperling L. Hair density in African Americans. Arch Dermatol 1999;135:656–8.

18. Bernstein RM, Rassman WR. The aesthetics of follicular transplantation. Dermatol Surg 1997;23:789–99.

19. Robles DT, Berg D. Abnormal wound healing: keloids. Clin Dermatol 2007;25:26–32.

20. Marcaine (bupivacaine hydrochloride) [package insert] (online). Lake Forest, IL: Hospira, Inc.

21. Abbasi G. Hair transplantation without postoperative edema. Hair Transplant Forum Int 2005; 15:149.

22. Drake LE, Dinehart SM, Goltz RW, et al. Guidelines of care for local and regional anesthesia in cutaneous surgery. J Am Acad Dermatol 1995;33:504–9.

23. Callender VD, Davis EC. Hair transplantation technique: a flexible blade for preparing curly hair grafts. Dermatol Surg 2011;37:1032–4.

24. Mathew AJ. A review of cellular biopreservation considerations during hair transplantation. Hair Transplant Forum Int 2013;23:1.

25. Davis EC, Reid SD, Callender VD, et al. Differentiating central centrifugal cicatricial alopecia and androgenetic alopecia in African-American men: report of 3 cases. J Clin Aesthet Dermatol 2012;5(6):37–40.

26. Callender V, Davis E. Hair transplantation. In: Alexis A, Barbosa VH, editors. Skin of color: a practical guide to dermatologic diagnosis and treatment. New York: Springer; 2013. p. 351–70.

27. Harris JA. New methodology and instrumentation for follicular unit extraction: lower follicle transection rates and expanded patient candidacy. Dermatol Surg 2006;32:56–61.

Central Centrifugal Cicatricial Alopecia
What Has Been Achieved, Current Clues for Future Research

Temitayo A. Ogunleye, MD[a],*, Amy McMichael, MD[b],
Elise A. Olsen, MD[c]

KEYWORDS

- Central centrifugal cicatricial alopecia • Hot comb alopecia • Scarring alopecia
- Follicular degeneration syndrome

KEY POINTS

- Central centrifugal cicatricial alopecia is a common condition that mostly affects women of African descent and may occur in families.
- The cause of central centrifugal cicatricial alopecia is unclear and current evidence does not support a strong causal association with traction and/or the use of relaxers.
- Because genetic predisposition may be unmasked by grooming, patients are advised to avoid or limit the use of relaxers, heat, and occlusive moisturizers.
- Studies are needed to provide evidence-based therapeutic regimens for this condition.

INTRODUCTION

Hair loss is a frequent complaint in women of African descent. In 1983, Halder and colleagues[1] described alopecia as the fifth most common dermatosis in African Americans, with chemical and traction alopecias being cited as the most common types. Since that time, central centrifugal cicatricial alopecia (CCCA), a lymphocyte mediated type of central scalp hair loss seen primarily in women of African descent, has been described with increasing frequency. Despite the prevalence of this condition, there has been a paucity of data on incidence, cause, and evidence-based therapeutic regimens. However, recent studies and literature are elucidating possible clues for future research for this seemingly enigmatic condition.

Before discussing in depth the specific condition of CCCA, it is worthwhile to review the specifics of hair and hair care practices unique to women of African descent.

HAIR MORPHOLOGY

Although there are no biochemical differences between hair of African, European, and Asian descent, hair morphology does differ.[2] Black hair appears elliptical in cross-section, with a curved follicle[3,4] and is in contrast to the oval-appearing follicle of Caucasians and round follicle of Asians.[3] African hair has a high degree of irregularity in the diameter along the hair shaft, with frequent twists and random reversals in direction.[3,4] It is also curlier and exhibits more knots, with decreased

Disclosure Statement: The authors have no relevant disclosures.
[a] Department of Dermatology, Perelman Center for Advanced Medicine, University of Pennsylvania, South Pavilion, 1st Floor, 3400 Civic Center Boulevard, Philadelphia, PA 19104, USA; [b] Department of Dermatology, Wake Forest Baptist Health, 4618 Country Club Road, Winston-Salem, NC 27104, USA; [c] Department of Dermatology, Hair Disorders Research and Treatment Center, Duke University Medical Center 3294, Durham, NC 27710, USA
* Corresponding author.
E-mail address: Temitayo.ogunleye@uphs.upenn.edu

Dermatol Clin 32 (2014) 173–181
http://dx.doi.org/10.1016/j.det.2013.12.005
0733-8635/14/$ – see front matter © 2014 Elsevier Inc. All rights reserved.

ability of sebum to coat the hair, leading to less shiny and drier hair[5,6]; this may be one factor contributing to African hair having less tensile strength and breaking more easily than Caucasian hair. In addition, studies suggest that overall hair density in black people may be less than that in Caucasians.[3] When comparing the biopsies of the scalp in 22 African Americans to 12 Caucasians without hair loss, Sperling[7] documented a lower hair density, with an average of 36 follicles per 4-mm-diameter round punch found in the Caucasian specimens compared with 22 follicles in the African American specimens. African hair has also been found to have fewer elastic fibers anchoring the hair follicles to the dermis.[8,9] These race-related differences in hair structure may play a role in the types of styling that black woman choose, and the subsequent development of CCCA.[10]

HAIR CARE PRACTICES

Black women can spend a great deal of time and money grooming their hair and may visit hair salons weekly or every 2 weeks for styling.[11] Straightening tends to be the styling method of choice, as it believed to lead to increased manageability, although other methods are used to increase styling options and flexibility in appearance.[12]

Methods of Straightening

Thermal straightening, also known as hot combing or pressing, was the first method used by African American women to straighten their hair. It was popularized by Madame CJ Walker in the 1900s after she developed a wide-tooth comb, making it feasible to comb African American hair. Thermal hair straightening is accomplished by temporarily rearranging hydrogen bonds within the hair shafts.[10] The process involves coating the hair with a lubricating oil or grease and combing the hair in sections with a very hot metal comb heated to 300 to 500°F until the hair has reached the desired level of straightness.[13] Although less popular today, many black women still use this thermal technique as an alternative method to chemical relaxing. In the large series of 529 African American women ages 18 to 85 reported by Olsen and colleagues[14] under the North American Hair Research Society (NAHRS) banner, 58% had ever used hot combs with 87% of those having used this by age 15 years old.

Flat irons are an alternative method of using heat as a method of hair straightening. Women place their hair between 2 smooth, often ceramic plates that are thought to heat more evenly and quickly than hot combs. Temperatures may still range from 180 to 450°F, but the even heating and better temperature control is thought to decrease potential damage. In addition, use of greases and oils is generally discouraged with this method, with many women using silicone-based heat protectant products to reduce damage to hair.

Alternate methods of hair straightening including the use of chemical relaxers were developed in the 1960s. The 2 major chemical agents used are sodium hydroxide in lye relaxers, and guanidine hydroxide found in no-lye relaxers. These hair relaxers produce permanent hair straightening by rearranging the disulfide bonds, accounting for the sulfurous odor sometimes noted during use. Relaxer use, in particularly when used improperly, has been associated with several adverse reactions, including irritant contact dermatitis, trichorrhexis nodosa, and brittle, more easily damaged hair.[15,16] This brittle nature of the hair is likely associated with the reduced cysteine content found in relaxer-treated hair, which is crucial for hair strength because it is a component of the disulfide bonds broken by the chemicals.[16] Chemical straightening via relaxers is currently much more popular than hot combing, with 90% of African American women having used this method at some point.[14]

Styling

Hairstyling with braids and weaves is popular in people of African descent. There are several methods for braiding hair, including braiding into sections to produce "cornrows," or adding human or synthetic hair for additional length and volume.[10] Weaving uses similar methods whereby the hair is cornrowed, and additional synthetic or human hair is sewn or glued to the base of the hair, and the additional hair is worn loose. "Locs" or dreadlocks are a type of styling that traditionally avoids chemical or heat processing and allows the hair to knot into individual twistlike structures. These structures can be maintained via twisting/ "palm-rolling" the root of the loc to allow for a uniform or "manicured" look (**Fig. 1**) or may be free-formed, such that the locs/dreadlocks are allowed to form with little to no intervention. This styling may lead to tension at the root of locs if they are overtwisted, if each section is too small, or if locs are allowed to grow to very long lengths. These methods of styling have been associated with traction alopecia[17] or marginal scalp hair loss, but because this type of styling is mostly unique to people of the African diaspora, there has been some speculation regarding their relationship to CCCA.

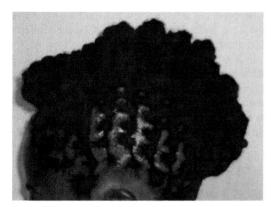

Fig. 1. Manicured locs in an elaborate style.

Hair Cleansing

African American women tend to shampoo less frequently than those of European descent, the most common frequency being once every 1 to 2 weeks.[11] Some hairstyling methods are costly and time-consuming, which may contribute to the relative infrequency of hair washing needed to maintain these styles.[4] In a study by Hall and colleagues,[11] 85% of women surveyed spent 0 to 5 hours at the salon at each visit, and 46% of the women spent greater than $50 monthly on hair care. In addition, most African American women studied wore their hair in a relaxed or straightened style, which reverts to a more native or curlier texture when wet.[11] The longevity of styles with weaves, braids, and locs may also be shortened by frequent shampooing. Last, shampooing too frequently may increase hair breakage secondary to decreasing relatively low levels of sebum on the hair shaft. How this infrequent removal of surface microorganisms may be related to CCCA remains to be evaluated.

HISTORY OF CCCA

This entity was first published in the literature by LoPresti and coworkers,[13] in 1968, whereby they described an "irreversible alopecia of the scalp" in black women in their 20s and 30s, with a characteristic course of beginning on the crown and spreading peripherally, sparing the lateral and posterior aspects of the scalp. This hair loss differed from that seen in other scarring conditions such as morphea or discoid lupus erythematosus, in that the skin remained soft and pliable, with a "glistening, shiny surface," although there was a "striking...decrease in the density of the follicular orifices."[13] They found that the 51 black women studied clinically with these findings all straightened their hair with hot combs, "in order to

conform with cosmetic standards of the fashion setting white group," although they describe one case with similar clinical findings in a Caucasian woman who had used a hot curling iron for years.[13] It was postulated that the hot petrolatum/oil used while hot combing ran down the hair shafts of the central scalp, causing a chronic lymphocytic inflammation around the upper segment of the hair follicle, leading to external root sheath degeneration, follicle destruction, and finally, follicular scarring. This entity was coined "hot comb alopecia."[13]

Following this description, there was little mention of this entity in the literature for over 2 decades except for occasional mentions in review articles on alopecia.[18,19] However, by 1987, Price[19] recognized that hot comb usage was not essential for development of the condition and recommended abandoning the term "hot comb alopecia." In 1992, Sperling and Sau[20] "revisited and revised" this condition. In their study 10 black women who were seeking evaluation of their central scalp hair loss were found to have histologic findings of premature desquamation of the inner root sheath, lamellar fibroplasia, and mononuclear inflammation, consistent with this condition. They found that not all patients had a history of hot comb use and that this method of styling was not temporally related to the onset or progression of this condition.[20] In addition, the use of hot combs had fallen in popularity by the early 1990s and had been somewhat replaced by the use of relaxers, yet cases of this condition persisted. Furthermore, patients in their control group of 10 women with no history of hair loss or hair problems practiced similar hair care methods (including use of hot combs and/or relaxers) and had not developed the entity. They proposed that "a predisposed population...exists that begins to express premature desquamation of the inner root sheath some time during adulthood."[20] Several factors, including mechanical factors specific to the follicle, heredity, and methods of hair grooming, contributed to this predisposition, and any combination of the above could lead to the expression of the syndrome.[20] They also noted that this condition does not seem to begin in childhood, so that the defect must emerge later in life, or be expressed in relation to certain factors such as traumatic hair care techniques.[20] Secondary to the seemingly specific histologic findings of premature inner root sheath degeneration and migration of the hair shaft through the outer root sheath, Sperling and Sau[20] proposed the term "follicular degeneration syndrome (FDS)."

In a 1996 review, Headington[21] argued that the follicular degeneration syndrome was not a distinct clinicopathologic entity but that the findings of selective premature degeneration of the follicular inner hair sheath may be seen in a variety of different scarring alopecias.[21] He postulated that premature fragmentation of the inner sheath is probably a result of altered outer hair sheath biology by cell-mediated injury or trauma. He used the term "scarring alopecia in African Americans" and proposed that a combination of relaxer use in addition to traction may contribute to the development of this condition.[21]

In 2000, Sperling and coworkes[22] coined the term central centrifugal scarring alopecia, to encompass clinical patterns of hair loss that have the following findings:

1. Hair loss centered on the crown or vertex of the scalp
2. Chronic and progressive disease with eventual burnout
3. Symmetric expansion with most active disease at the periphery
4. Both clinical and histologic evidence of inflammation in the active peripheral zone.

By this definition, central centrifugal scarring alopecia included not only follicular degeneration syndrome, but other conditions, such as traumatic alopecia, folliculitis decalvans, lichen planopilaris, or discoid lupus erythematosus.

In 2001, the term "central centrifugal cicatricial alopecia (CCCA)" was adopted by the NAHRS to refer specifically to the central scarring hair loss seen predominately in African Americans. This term encompassed hot comb alopecia and follicular degeneration syndrome.[23]

CLINICAL FEATURES

The clinical features of CCCA that have been described have remained constant over the decades. Patients present with a chronic and progressive central scalp hair loss that expands centrifugally in a somewhat symmetric fashion.[14] Advanced cases show a smooth and shiny scalp with impressive follicular dropout. Occasionally, a few strands of hair remain in the affected bald area, some demonstrating polytrichia. There is typically no overt evidence of inflammation,[24] although there may be erythema or follicular pustules early in the course.[25] However, follicular erythema or papules as seen with lichen planopilaris are lacking (**Fig. 2A–C**).

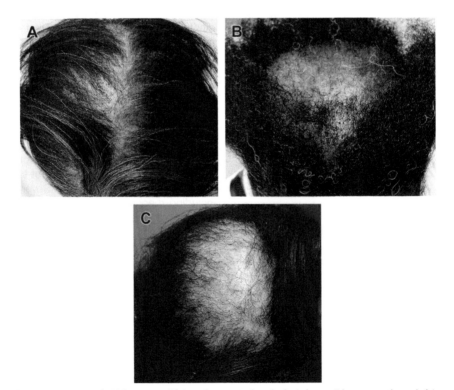

Fig. 2. (A–C) Various stages of CCCA exemplifying the central scalp hair loss with a smooth and shiny scalp with impressive follicular dropout. Note the few strands that commonly remain in the affected area and the lack of inflammation.

Hair breakage has recently been described as a possible key early sign of early CCCA in a subset of patients. A recent retrospective study by Callender and colleagues[26] describes 9 patients who presented with hair breakage of the vertex of the scalp. Of the 8 biopsies performed in the affected area of the scalp that were evaluated by both vertical and horizontal sectioning, 5 demonstrated histologic changes characteristic of CCCA, including premature desquamation of the inner root sheath, concentric lamellar fibroplasia and perifollicular lymphocytic inflammation, but with varying degrees of severity.[26] Because the differential diagnosis of hair breakage is broad and typically associated with traumatic hair practices that are similarly found in patients with CCCA, a causative relationship is unclear. More studies are needed to determine the frequency of this clinical finding.

Symptoms may be nonexistent or notable with itching, tenderness, or burning in the areas of involvement. Bin Saif and colleagues[27] found that cowhage-induced itch, and not histamine-induced itch, correlates to CCCA severity ratings. Cowhage may serve as an adequate experimental model for scalp itch in CCCA.[27] These spicules stimulate protease-activated receptor-2 in the skin, which is a well-known mediator of chronic pruritus.[28] These findings suggest that protease-activated receptor-2 may play a role in the pathogenesis of CCCA, or at least may be a therapeutic target for these patients and elucidates an area of further study.[27]

However, because of the lack of symptoms in some patients, the condition may progress insidiously, leading to late presentation of the patient for medical care. One study found that hair stylists were responsible for alerting 21% of study patients about their hair loss.[24] Involvement is slow and progressive and can proceed to involve the entire central scalp (Fig. 3).

HISTOPATHOLOGY

Early histologic changes demonstrate a perifollicular lymphocytic infiltrate and perifollicular fibroplasia. This inflammatory infiltrate extends from the lower follicular infundibulum down to the upper isthmus. Terminal hair follicles reduction is noted with an increase in fibrous tracts. Premature desquamation of the inner root sheath (PDIRS) is one of the most important histologic markers of the disease, but is not specific to this condition and can be seen in other primary scarring alopecias.[21,29] Late-stage findings are indistinguishable from those found in other primary scarring alopecias, such as destruction of pilosebaceous units,

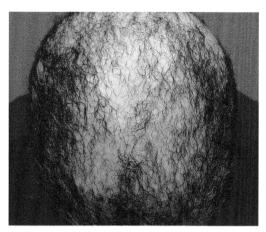

Fig. 3. Severe CCCA with nearly total scalp involvement.

dermal scarring, and dermal lymphocytic and plasma cell infiltrate.[21]

A recent study by Sperling and colleagues[30] examined cytokeratin 75 expression in affected and unaffected tissue. Cytokeratin 75 is expressed in the companion layer of the hair follicle, which lies between the outer and inner root sheaths. They found decreased expression of this keratin in relation to desquamation of the inner root sheath, occurring more prematurely (below the level of the isthmus) in CCCA follicles in comparison with normal follicles. However, they also found that expression in unaffected follicles in patients with CCCA was indistinguishable from that in normal follicles, suggesting that cytokeratin 75 expression may only highlight PDIRS and may not be directly involved in the pathogenesis of CCCA.[30] Further immunohistochemical studies such as these may serve to elucidate possible heritable or acquired mutations that predispose certain populations to CCCA.

EPIDEMIOLOGY

There is little epidemiologic data about CCCA. The condition has been presumed to occur primarily in women of African descent, since the reports described by LoPresti and colleagues[13] and Sperling and Sau.[20] In 1994, Sperling and Sau described a series of 8 black men who had clinical-pathologic findings consistent with follicular degeneration syndrome, but there are little other published data to support a large cohort of men of African descent with this disorder.[31] In addition, the patients in this series had more inflammatory disease than is commonly described in patients with CCCA, casting doubt on whether this is the same disease process. Case series and anecdotal evidence seem to support that this is a condition that primarily occurs in women of African descent.[32] In the Baylor Hair Research and Treatment Center, Whiting and Olsen[25] noted an average age of presentation of this condition of 36 years in women.

The prevalence of this condition in women of African descent is largely unknown. A recent study of the NAHRS published by Olsen and colleagues[14] in 2011 found that in 233 African American women evaluated in 3 randomly selected church group meetings where hair loss was specifically not discussed before the meetings, a hair loss pattern consistent with CCCA, but not histologically confirmed, occurred in 5.6% of women with a mean age of 48 years. Socioeconomic factors were not taken into account. Similarly, in a cross-sectional study by Khumalo[33] only 2.7% (but 6.7% >50 years of age) of the 604 black African women examined from church groups, community organizations, and hostels in Langa Township in South Africa had clinical, but not histologically confirmed evidence of CCCA. However, not surprisingly, a higher incidence (15.4%) of CCCA (confirmed histologically) was seen in a small Nigerian cross-sectional clinic study of 39 female patients seeking medical advice for hair loss.[34] More information is needed regarding variability in incidence in different countries of the African diaspora.

CAUSE

Hot combs were the first suspected etiologic agent as described by LoPresti in 1968,[13] but was later dismissed.[20] However, the belief that hair care practices affect an underlying predisposition to develop CCCA is largely accepted.

Hair Care Practices

Thus far, few studies have verified any direct correlation between hair care practices and the development of CCCA. The NAHRS study of 529 women found no statistically significant correlation between relaxer, hot comb, or texturizer use, or style with braided extension or weaves.[14] In the Kyei and colleagues'[35] publication of the Cleveland Clinic results of the NAHRS study, there was again no significant correlation between relaxer use or texturizer use, although a positive correlation of more severe grades of CCCA to traction-inducing hairstyles such as braids and weaves was found. A cross-sectional study by Khumalo and colleagues,[36] found that the prevalence of traction alopecia was highest (48%) when weaves/braids were attached to relaxed hair, suggesting that combining different styling techniques may worsen hair loss. However,

reanalysis of the data from the 604 women in this study[36] with data from 574 schoolgirls[37] did not reveal any significant associations between CCCA and relaxer use or traction-inducing hairstyles. In the Gathers and colleagues[24] study, a retrospective comparative survey comparing 51 women with clinical and histologic diagnosis of CCCA and a control group of 50 women without a diagnosis of alopecia found no correlation between the use of either hot combing and hair relaxers to CCCA. However, a significant association was found between the use of both sew-in hair weaves and braided styles with CCCA.[24]

Female Pattern Hair Loss

In 2003 and 2005, Olsen described a theory that CCCA may begin as female pattern hair loss (FPHL), which is then adversely affected by hair care practices.[38,39] There is support for this theory given that in the NAHRS study,[14] there was an increase in patterns I and II central hair loss that are clinically consistent with FPHL, consistent with that seen in Caucasian women (Olsen EA, unpublished information, personal communication, 2013). That CCCA may begin as an androgen-dependent process is also supported by the high incidence of hirsutism (48%) and irregular periods (24%) in the larger group of 529 African American women in the NAHRS study, findings which were unrelated to any pattern of hair loss (Olsen EA, unpublished information, personal communication, 2013). The NAHRS group is now embarking on a study to merge clinical and laboratory features with biopsy findings in African American women with this condition, which should provide data around the relatedness of FPHL and CCCA.

The Role of Chronic Inflammation and Microorganisms

The inner root sheath acts as a seal for the noncornified portion of the hair follicle from the infundibular portion.[30] Cytokines extracted from scalp sebum were reported to suggest a pro-inflammatory state even in women with natural hair (IL-1α18 times higher than IL-1 receptor antagonist).[40] It has been postulated that if PDIRS is the primary event that occurs in CCCA, then external material such as cosmetics and microorganisms could reach lower portions of the follicle, leading to chronic inflammation and eventual scarring.[30] Thus, the common greases and occlusive moisturizers used frequently by African American women could increase the growth of microorganisms through occlusion. In fact, in the NAHRS study, one of the key findings was the relatively high incidence of tinea capitis in African American women with extensive central hair loss.[14] They did not, however, find any difference in reports of bacterial infections between those with minimal (patterns I and II) and those with extensive (patterns III-V) central scalp hair loss.[14] Also, the reports of both tinea capitis and bacterial infection were all based on patient recall and not documented infection.

Family History

A genetic predisposition or family history of this condition has more recently been examined a possible strong risk factor. In the Olsen and colleagues[14] NAHRS cross-sectional study, family history of similar hair loss in the patient's mother was found to be statistically significant. In the Kyei and colleagues'[35] publication of the Cleveland Clinic results of the larger NAHRS study, they found that there was a statistically significant increase in central hair loss in the maternal grandfather among those who had more severe grades of CCCA. In a recent 2012 report, Dlova and Forder[41] found evidence of familial cause in 2 South African families. One family examined revealed 4 siblings, ages 45, 55, 63, and 65 years old, and their 92-year-old mother with clinical and histologic evidence of CCCA. Biopsies demonstrated eccentric thinning of the follicular epithelium with concentric lamellar fibroplasia, even though the mother had no reported history of any chemical or mechanical trauma. Another family included a 35-year-old mother and her 11-year-old daughter who also had clinical and histologic evidence of CCCA. The 11-year-old daughter also had no history of chemical or mechanical trauma to her hair. Of note, affected family members in both families who had a frequent history of braids, weaves, or relaxer use seemed to exhibit more severe phenotypes than those with "virgin" hair or infrequent use of these styling practices. These findings may suggest that there may be a genetic defect in the internal root sheath in some Africans or African Americans as a primary pathologic event,[41] or a common environmental exposure, such as shared hair care practices or a combination of both. Aggravation or triggering of the disease may occur with traumatic hair care practices.[41] Further studies are necessary to confirm this interesting observation.

TREATMENT

There are no published case-controlled studies documenting effective treatment of CCCA, although there are many anecdotal reports of successes. Treatments are mostly aimed at medical anti-inflammatory therapy, with surgical therapies being the only option in very late end-stage disease. Realistic expectations for therapy should include stopping the progression of the condition,[10] as well as relieving symptoms, with any hair regrowth noted to be an added bonus. Despite lack of strong evidence directly associating hair care practices, removal of potentially damaging hair-care practices is encouraged, including increased intervals between relaxer applications (every 8–10 weeks), decreased use of heat to the scalp, and decrease in the tightness of weaves and braids.[10] A seborrheic dermatitis regimen may be helpful in decreasing itching and scaling. Topical and intralesional steroids are first-line therapy at some centers.[42] Topical steroids are used daily until symptoms abate and then are tapered to 3 days per week for maintenance. Intralesional steroids ranging in strength from 2.5 to 10 mg/mL may be used every 4 to 8 weeks, for a period of at least 6 months.[10,24,42] The target area should be at the periphery of areas of hair loss, including surrounding areas of normal-appearing scalp to prevent progression.[43]

Other anti-inflammatory treatments including oral tetracyclines and antimalarials have been used with varying success.[44] Treatments including minoxidil, thalidomide, mycophenolate mofetil, vitamins, and cyclosporine have been suggested, but are not commonly used.[4,45] Treatments usually are sustained for at least 6 months until remission is obtained, although they may need to be restarted for any flares that may occur.[43] Olsen has used anti-androgens and/or 5-α-reductase inhibitors with success (unpublished information, personal communication, 2013).

Surgical correction via hair transplantation is a possible option for patients with this condition. As with any scarring form of hair loss involving inflammation, it is important to make sure that the infiltrate is no longer active before hair restoration, as there could be destruction of grafts by the infiltrates. Occurrence of disfiguring keloids occurs at a fairly low frequency, despite common fears.[10] When performed correctly, black patients tend to have the appearance of denser growth secondary to the curly nature of the hair.[46,47] However, hair transplantation in this condition tends to be more complicated secondary to the scarring of the recipient site inherent to this condition, and the decrease in the survival rate of the transplanted grafts.[10]

CURRENT CLUES FOR FUTURE RESEARCH

Since this condition was first described by LoPresti and colleagues[13] in 1968, the cause of this condition remains a mystery. Although hot combs and relaxers have been proven not to be a primary causative agent, it is still likely that hair care practices used by African American women play a role in the pathogenesis of CCCA, providing an opportunity for further population-based studies. As popular methods of styling shift according to changes in cultural norms, it will also be interesting to note if the "natural" (avoidance of chemical means of straightening) movement will decrease the seemingly high prevalence of this condition in the next few years.

The role of genetics/heredity is another potential area of study, especially with recent reports of familial cases in patients with no history of traumatic hair care practices. Further immunohistochemical/pathologic studies examining the inner root sheath and the events that lead to its desquamation are necessary. In addition, randomized controlled studies examining the efficacy of treatments to reduce the progression and the symptoms associated with the condition are lacking and are a necessary addition to the literature. After over a 20-year lack of research or publications about CCCA since it was first described, there seems to be a welcome renewed interest in the condition, and in unlocking the mystery behind the pathogenesis of this relatively common and progressive condition.

REFERENCES

1. Halder RM, Grimes PE, McLaurin CI, et al. Incidence of common dermatoses in a predominantly black dermatologic practice. Cutis 1983;32(4):388–90.

2. Lindelof B, Forslind B, Hedblad MA, et al. Human hair form. Morphology revealed by light and scanning electron microscopy and computer aided three-dimensional reconstruction. Arch Dermatol 1988;124(9):1359–63.

3. Franbourg A, Hallegot P, Baltenneck F, et al. Current research on ethnic hair. J Am Acad Dermatol 2003; 48(Suppl 6):S115–9.

4. McMichael AJ. Ethnic hair update: past and present. J Am Acad Dermatol 2003;48(Suppl 6):S127–33.

5. Khumalo NP, Doe PT, Dawber RP, et al. What is normal black African hair? A light and scanning electron-microscopic study. J Am Acad Dermatol 2000;43(5 Pt 1):814–20.

6. Johnson BA. Requirements in cosmetics for black skin. Dermatol Clin 1988;6(3):489–92.

7. Sperling LC. Hair density in African Americans. Arch Dermatol 1999;135(6):656–8.

8. Taylor S. Practical tips for managing hair disorders in African-American females. Przegl Dermatol 2006; 3(7):25–7.

9. Richards GM, Oresajo CO, Halder RM. Structure and function of ethnic skin and hair. Dermatol Clin 2003;21(4):595–600.

10. Callender VD, McMichael AJ, Cohen GF. Medical and surgical therapies for alopecias in black women. Dermatol Ther 2004;17(2):164–76.

11. Hall RR, Francis S, Whitt-Glover M, et al. Hair care practices as a barrier to physical activity in African American women. JAMA Dermatol 2013;149(3): 310–4.

12. Callendar V. African-American scalp disorders and treatment considerations. Skin Aging 2002; 10(Suppl):12–4.

13. LoPresti P, Papa CM, Kligman AM. Hot comb alopecia. Arch Dermatol 1968;98(3):234–8.

14. Olsen EA, Callender V, McMichael A, et al. Central hair loss in African American women: incidence and potential risk factors. J Am Acad Dermatol 2011;64(2):245–52.

15. Swee W, Klontz KC, Lambert LA. A nationwide outbreak of alopecia associated with the use of a hair-relaxing formulation. Arch Dermatol 2000; 136(9):1104–8.

16. Khumalo NP, Stone J, Gumedze F, et al. "Relaxers" damage hair: evidence from amino acid analysis. J Am Acad Dermatol 2010;62(3):402–8.

17. Grimes PE. Skin and hair cosmetic issues in women of color. Dermatol Clin 2000;18(4):659–65.

18. Whiting D. Current concepts: the diagnosis of alopecia. Kalamazoo (MI): The Upjohn Co; 1990. p. 24.

19. Price V. Hair loss in cutaneous disease. In: Baden HP, editor. Symposium on Alopecia. New York: HP Publishing Co; 1987.

20. Sperling LC, Sau P. The follicular degeneration syndrome in black patients. "Hot comb alopecia" revisited and revised. Arch Dermatol 1992;128(1):68–74.

21. Headington JT. Cicatricial alopecia. Dermatol Clin 1996;14(4):773–82.

22. Sperling LC, Solomon AR, Whiting DA. A new look at scarring alopecia. Arch Dermatol 2000;136(2): 235–42.

23. Olsen EA, Bergfeld WF, Cotsarelis G, et al. Summary of North American Hair Research Society (NAHRS)-sponsored Workshop on Cicatricial Alopecia, Duke University Medical Center, February 10 and 11, 2001. J Am Acad Dermatol 2003;48(1):103–10.

24. Gathers RC, Jankowski M, Eide M, et al. Hair grooming practices and central centrifugal cicatricial alopecia. J Am Acad Dermatol 2009;60(4):574–8.

25. Whiting DA, Olsen EA. Central centrifugal cicatricial alopecia. Dermatol Ther 2008;21(4):268–78.

26. Callender VD, Wright DR, Davis EC, et al. Hair breakage as a presenting sign of early or occult central centrifugal cicatricial alopecia: clinicopathologic findings in 9 patients. Arch Dermatol 2012;148(9): 1047–52.

27. Bin Saif GA, McMichael A, Kwatra SG, et al. Central centrifugal cicatricial alopecia severity is associated with cowhage-induced itch. Br J Dermatol 2013; 168(2):253–6.

28. Bin Saif GA, Ericson ME, Yosipovitch G. The itchy scalp–scratching for an explanation. Exp Dermatol 2011;20(12):959–68.

29. Whiting DA. Cicatricial alopecia: clinicopathological findings and treatment. Clin Dermatol 2001;19: 211–5.

30. Sperling LC, Hussey S, Sorrells T, et al. Cytokeratin 75 expression in central, centrifugal, cicatricial alopecia–new observations in normal and diseased hair follicles. J Cutan Pathol 2010;37(2):243–8.

31. Sperling LC, Skelton HG 3rd, Smith KJ, et al. Follicular degeneration syndrome in men. Arch Dermatol 1994;130(6):763–9.

32. Shah SK, Alexis AF. Central centrifugal cicatricial alopecia: retrospective chart review. J Cutan Med Surg 2010;14(5):212–22.

33. Khumalo NP. Prevalence of central centrifugal cicatricial alopecia. Arch Dermatol 2011;147(12):1453–4 [author reply: 1454].

34. Nnoruka EN. Hair loss: is there a relationship with hair care practices in Nigeria? Int J Dermatol 2005; 44(Suppl 1):13–7.

35. Kyei A, Bergfeld WF, Piliang M, et al. Medical and environmental risk factors for the development of central centrifugal cicatricial alopecia: a population study. Arch Dermatol 2011;147(8):909–14.

36. Khumalo NP, Jessop S, Gumedze F, et al. Hairdressing and the prevalence of scalp disease in African adults. Br J Dermatol 2007;157(5):981–8.

37. Khumalo NP, Jessop S, Gumedze F. Hairdressing is associated with scalp disease in African schoolchildren. Br J Dermatol 2007;157:106–10.

38. Olsen E. Pattern hair loss. In: Olsen EA, editor. Disorders of hair growth: diagnosis and treatment. New York: McGraw-Hill; 2003. p. 326.

39. Olsen EA. Female pattern hair loss and its relationship to permanent/cicatricial alopecia: a new perspective. J Investig Dermatol Symp Proc 2005; 10(3):217–21.

40. Beach RA, Wilkinson KA, Gumedze F, et al. Baseline sebum IL-1α is higher than expected in afro-textured hair: a risk factor for hair loss? J Cosmet Dermatol 2012;11(1):9–16.

41. Dlova NC, Forder M. Central centrifugal cicatricial alopecia: possible familial aetiology in two African families from South Africa. Int J Dermatol 2012; 51(Suppl 1):17–20, 20–3.

42. Gathers RC, Lim HW. Central centrifugal cicatricial alopecia: past, present, and future. J Am Acad Dermatol 2009;60(4):660–8.

43. McMichael AJ, Hordinsky M, editors. Hair diseases: medical, surgical, and cosmetic treatments. New York: Informa USA; 2008.

44. McMichael AJ. Scalp and hair disorders in African-American patients: a primer of disorders and treatments. J Cosmet Dermatol 2003;16:37–41.

45. Price VH. The medical treatment of cicatricial alopecia. Semin Cutan Med Surg 2006;25(1):56–9.

46. Unger W. Hair transplantation in blacks. In: Unger W, editor. Hair transplantation. New York: Marcel Dekker; 1995. p. 281–5.

47. Pierce HE. The uniqueness of hair transplantation in black patients. J Dermatol Surg Oncol 1977;3(5): 533–5.

Folliculitis Keloidalis Nuchae and Pseudofolliculitis Barbae

Are Prevention and Effective Treatment Within Reach?

Andrew Alexis, MD, MPH[a],*, Candrice R. Heath, MD[b],
Rebat M. Halder, MD[c]

KEYWORDS

- Folliculitis keloidalis nuchae • Pseudofolliculitis barbae • Acne keloidalis nuchae • Razor bumps
- Ingrown hairs • Ethnic skin • Skin of color

KEY POINTS

- Pseudofolliculitis barbae (PFB) is an inflammatory follicular disorder associated with shaving, most commonly seen in men of African ancestry.
- Follicular penetration from ingrown hairs is the primary inciting factor in PFB.
- In the appropriate patient, an effective prevention strategy for PFB is to grow a beard, but optimization of shaving practices (including pre- and postcare) is a useful approach for men who wish to continue shaving.
- Folliculitis keloidalis nuchae (FKN) is a follicular-based disorder mainly affecting the nape of the neck; histopathologically, FKN has characteristics of a primary cicatricial alopecia.
- PFB and FKN are chronic conditions requiring continual maintenance strategies.

INTRODUCTION

Pseudofolliculitis barbae (PFB) and folliculitis keloidalis nuchae (FKN) are chronic follicular disorders that disproportionally affect men of African ancestry. Though common, these conditions are often therapeutically challenging, requiring pharmacologic, procedural, and behavioral approaches to treatment. In this article the epidemiology, pathogenesis, clinical findings, treatment options, prevention, and new advances with regard to PFB and FKN are discussed. The possibility of achieving effective preventive measures and treatments is also explored.

PSEUDOFOLLICULITIS BARBAE
Epidemiology

PFB is a common follicular disorder most prevalent in men of African ancestry.[1–3] It is also frequently observed among Hispanic, Middle Eastern, and other populations in whom tightly curled hair is common. Among African American men, the incidence of PFB is 45% to 83%.[4–6]

Disclosure: Actual or potential conflict of interest, including employment, consultancies, stock ownership, patent applications/registrations, grants, other funding. A. Alexis: Consulting (Allergan, Galderma, L'Oreal USA, Schick); C.R. Heath: none; R.M. Halder: Consulting (L'Oreal USA, Combe Corporation, KCI), Grants (L'Oreal USA).

[a] Department of Dermatology, Skin of Color Center, St. Luke's-Roosevelt Hospital, 1090 Amsterdam Avenue, Suite 11 B, New York, NY 10025, USA; [b] Department of Dermatology, St. Luke's-Roosevelt Hospital Center, 1090 Amsterdam Avenue, Suite 11 B, New York, NY 10025, USA; [c] Department of Dermatology, Howard University College of Medicine, 2041 Georgia Avenue, Northwest, Washington, DC 20060, USA
* Corresponding author.
E-mail address: alexisderm@yahoo.com

Dermatol Clin 32 (2014) 183–191
http://dx.doi.org/10.1016/j.det.2013.12.001
0733-8635/14/$ – see front matter © 2014 Elsevier Inc. All rights reserved.

PFB may also occur in any race and may also affect women.[1,7,8]

Pathogenesis

PFB is a chronic, noninfectious inflammatory disorder resulting from a foreign-body reaction to the hair shaft. Individuals who have coarse, tightly curled hair and who shave are predisposed to this condition, owing to the tendency for the distal portion of tightly curled hair shafts to reenter the skin after shaving. Reentry of shaved hair shafts can occur through 1 of 2 mechanisms: (1) extrafollicular penetration, whereby the shaved hair shaft grows along its natural curvature and penetrates the epidermis 1 to 2 mm distal to the follicular opening; or (2) transfollicular penetration, whereby the sharp distal tip of a shaved hair shaft retracts beneath the skin surface, pierces the follicular wall, and enters the dermis. Stretching the skin during shaving or close shaving techniques can contribute to transfollicular penetration.[4,9,10]

Hair reentry (via either extrafollicular or transfollicular penetration) results in a chronic, foreign-body inflammatory response.[1] In addition to this mechanical etiology, a genetic risk factor has been identified that can affect a subset of men with PFB. A substitution mutation in the 1A α-helical segment of the hair-follicle–specific keratin 75 (formerly K6hf) was found in 36% of PFB cases compared with 9% in controls ($P<.000006$). This single nucleotide polymorphism may be associated with a structurally weakened companion layer of the hair follicle which, along with curly hair shafts and close shaving, contributes to an increased risk for PFB.[11]

Clinical Features

The clinical hallmarks of PFB are follicular and/or perifollicular papules in an area where repetitive shaving has occurred (**Fig. 1**). In men, the most commonly affected area is the neck (**Fig. 2**) followed by the cheeks, whereas in women the chin (especially the submental region) is the most commonly affected area.[4] Of note, the moustache and nuchal areas are rarely affected. Hirsute women who shave or pluck unwanted hairs frequently develop PFB on the chin and neck area (**Fig. 3**). Shaving the axillae and bikini region of the groin, a common practice among women of all races, can lead to pseudofolliculitis in these areas.[7]

The papules of PFB may be firm, skin colored, erythematous, or hyperpigmented. If secondary infection arises, pustules and papulopustules may be present.[8] Some papules may contain visible hairs.[3] Linear depressions in the affected

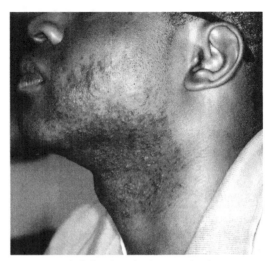

Fig. 1. Pseudofolliculitis barbae with characteristic perifollicular papules and pustules on the beard area. Note the associated postinflammatory hyperpigmentation.

skin areas likely represent hairs that are growing parallel to the surface of the skin (**Fig. 4**).[4] Potential sequelae include postinflammatory hyperpigmentation (PIH) and keloids.[1] Pruritus and pain are also potential associated clinical features.[3,8]

The differential diagnosis of PFB includes acne vulgaris, sycosis barbae, and traumatic folliculitis. No comedonal lesions are found in PFB, and acne vulgaris affects other areas of the face in addition to the beard area. Pustules are common in acne vulgaris, whereas they are rare in PFB. In sycosis barbae, perifollicular pustules are the primary and predominant lesions. Lesions in PFB are isolated, whereas in sycosis barbae they are confluent. Shaving improves sycosis barbae, whereas it makes PFB worse. Traumatic folliculitis, commonly known as razor burn, occurs when shaving is done too closely. Lesions are erythematous, painful, small follicular papules, which disappear within 24 to 48 hours after shaving.

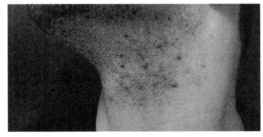

Fig. 2. Pseudofolliculitis barbae involving the neck (the most common region affected in men with this disorder).

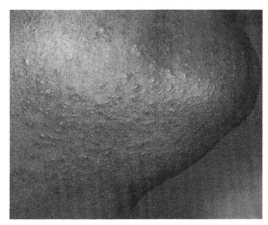

Fig. 3. Pseudofolliculitis barbae involving the chin and submental region in a woman with hirsutism who tweezed and shaved unwanted hairs.

Pseudofolliculitis barbae persists for several weeks after cessation of shaving.

Management

The goal of PFB management is to improve the cosmetic appearance of the affected area, enhance one's self-esteem, appropriately address impacts of PFB on occupational requirements, and prevent further complications such as hypertrophic scarring, keloidal scarring, or infection.

Setting reasonable expectations regarding potential treatment outcomes is a priority. PFB is a chronic problem for which the only true cure is growing a beard or having the hairs permanently removed.[12]

Many patients are disturbed by the appearance of PFB lesions. Not only do these lesions potentially impact self-esteem, they may also lead to an inability to comply with workplace

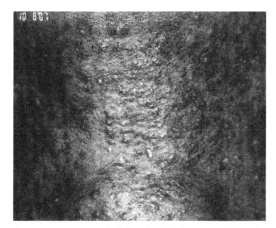

Fig. 4. Severe pseudofolliculitis barbae involving the neck. Note coarse hair shafts growing tangentially on the upper third of the neck.

grooming policies. Men working in jobs requiring a close-shaven appearance may experience personal distress, along with repercussions from employers. Occupations such as flight attendant, police officer, and food service worker often require a close shave. African Americans in the military are often forced to choose between worsening their PFB with close shaves or be at risk for discharge from the armed forces.[4,5,13,14]

Treatment options for PFB are summarized in **Table 1**. The initial consultation for a patient with PFB should begin with a detailed discussion of therapeutic options and can involve a stepwise approach (**Fig. 5**). The first step is offering the patient the option of growing a beard, as discontinuation of shaving for at least 1 month has been shown to be curative in most cases. Patients who choose this option may require a physician letter for their employer to permit them to maintain a well-groomed beard in their professional setting. For patients who prefer not to have a beard, recommendations are directed toward minimization of hair shaft reentry and reduction of inflammation. Modification of shaving practices, including the addition of preshave and postshave regimens, is helpful in achieving these goals. Before shaving, the beard area should be prepped by washing with warm water and a mild soap-free cleanser. Using a wash cloth or polyester cleansing pad in a circular motion is a helpful technique aimed at gently releasing embedded hair shafts before shaving. Preshave washing regimens (using a scrub or brush) have been shown to reduce the percentage of trapped beard hairs.[15] Shaving should be performed with a clean, sharp razor with the skin in its relaxed state (stretching of the skin should be avoided, as this may facilitate transfollicular penetration of hairs shaved slightly below the skin surface). Shaving in the direction of hair growth (ie, with the grain) has been generally recommended[4]; however, a recently published study found that men who reported shaving against the grain had lower papule counts.[16] Traditionally, single-blade razors have been favored over multiple-blade razors because of concerns about transfollicular penetration associated with the closer shave achieved with multiple-blade razors. However, in a recent study, PFB was not exacerbated by the use of multiple-blade razors (in conjunction with a preshave cleanser and postshave lotion).[16] Regardless of choice of a single-blade or multiple-blade razor, a clean, sharp razor blade should be used for each and every shave. Published comparative studies of single-blade versus multiple-blade razors or electric versus manual razors in patients with PFB are currently lacking, as are studies that

Table 1
Treatment options for pseudofolliculitis barbae (PFB) and folliculitis keloidalis nuchae (FKN)

Pharmacologic	Procedural
PFB Treatment Options	
Topical retinoids • Keratolytic[20] • Treats concomitant PIH[1,2,22] *Low- to mid-potency topical corticosteroids* • Anti-inflammatory[1,2,8] *Intralesional corticosteroids*[1,2,8] *Topical antibiotics*[19] • Antimicrobial[4] • Anti-inflammatory[19] *Bleaching creams for concomitant PIH* • Hydroquinone, kojic acid, azelaic acid[1–4,8] *Chemical depilatories* *Hair growth reduction* • Eflornithine hydrochloride cream 13.8%[27]	*Electrolysis/epilation* • Potential complications: tedious; needle may not go deep enough to destroy hair bulb[8] *Surgical depilation* • Permanent hair removal, via submandibular excision, hair bulbs electrodesiccated, extracted, or clipped[21] • Potential complications: expensive; keloid scarring in those prone to keloids in[8,21] *Punch excision*[8,18] *Chemical peels*[1–4,8,22] *Lasers* • Diode[24] • Long-pulse Nd:YAG[16,25] • Potential complications: dyspigmentation, scarring, blistering
FKN Treatment Options	
Corticosteroids (topical, intralesional), Class I or II corticosteroid gel or foam BID[43]	Removal with trephine device and secondary-intention healing/primary closure[28] Excision of nodules with tissue-expansion mechanisms[8,18] Laser[48,49]
Antibiotics (oral) tetracycline derivatives or topical clindamycin for secondary infection[1–3]	Excision with primary closure[46] Excision with healing by secondary intention[44]
Corticosteroid gel combined with retinoic acid gel[28]	Electrosurgical excision and secondary-intention healing[45] Cryotherapy[28]

Abbreviations: BID, twice daily; Nd:YAG, neodymium:yttrium aluminum garnet; PIH, postinflammatory hyperpigmentation.

prospectively investigate the effects of shaving direction on PFB severity.

Electrical razors are useful in controlling PFB, maintaining beard hair at an optimum length of 0.5 to 1 mm to prevent both transfollicular and extrafollicular penetration. Triple-O electric clippers can be used in this regard. These clippers have a protective gap between the comb-like projection that touches the skin and actual razor that cuts the hair. The success of electric clippers in controlling PFB has been impressive. However, clippers leave hair that is approximately 1 mm in length, and the appearance of the remaining stubble may not be acceptable to some patients.

A foil-guarded manual razor was developed for the treatment of PFB.[17] This razor has a single-edged, polymer-coated, stainless-steel blade with a serrated foil guard covering about 30% of its cutting edge. This guard acts as a partial buffer between the sharp blade and the skin, thus preventing hairs from being cut too close and causing transfollicular penetration. Reported results of shaving with this razor indicate improvement in most patients.

The judicious use of chemical depilatories (eg, barium sulfide powder or calcium thioglycolate cream formulations) can be a viable alternative to shaving. Barium sulfide depilatories give a smoother shave than calcium thioglycolate depilatories, but are less preferred because of malodor. However, irritant contact dermatitis and erosions are potential limitations. Prolonged contact time should be avoided to reduce the risk of irritation. A recent 1-week, split-faced, randomized trial comparing 3 depilatory formulations with shaving with a manual razor found that the depilatory compositions produced fewer papules than the manual razor, but postshaving irritation was more common with the depilatories.[18]

Pharmacologic treatments for PFB include low-potency topical corticosteroids (eg, desonide lotion), benzoyl peroxide formulations, topical antibiotics, and topical retinoids. Topical corticosteroids can be used for more severe cases, and

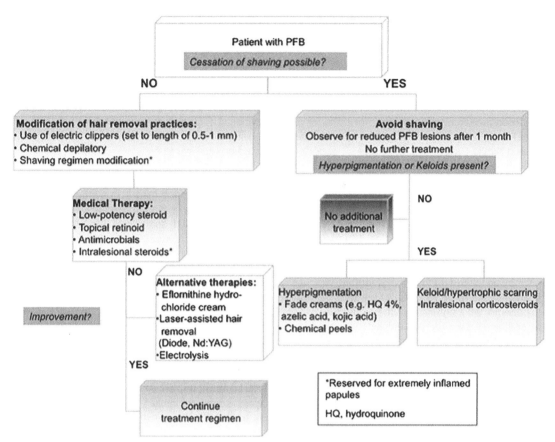

Fig. 5. Treatment algorithm for pseudofolliculitis barbae. (*From* Coley MK, Kelly AP, Alexis AF. Pseudofolliculitis barbae and acne keloidalis nuchae. In: Alexis AF, Barbosa VH, editors. Skin of color: a practical guide to dermatologic diagnosis and treatment, 1st edition. New York: Springer; 2013. p. 127; with permission.)

should generally be limited to 2-week courses or used 1 to 3 times per week to minimize risk of atrophy and other side effects. Benzoyl peroxide can be used alone or as a fixed combination with an antibiotic, and is recommended after shaving. The potential to bleach shirt collars is a possible limitation that should be conveyed to the patient. In a multicenter, double-blind, vehicle-controlled study, benzoyl peroxide 5%/clindamycin 1% gel demonstrated significant reductions in combined papule and pustule counts.[19] Topical retinoids (tretinoin, adapalene, or tazarotene) are recommended nightly, and are useful for improving both the clinical lesions of PFB[4,20,21] and the associated postinflammatory hyperpigmentation.[22] Postinflammatory hyperpigmentation can be a significant sequela in PFB, and can cause as much distress to the patient as do the primary lesions of PFB. Thus, bleaching preparations including hydroquinone can also be used for secondary postinflammatory hyperpigmentation.

For cases resistant to topical therapy or for patients with PFB who prefer a longer-term clean-shaven appearance, laser hair removal is an effective option.[23–25] Using lasers that are safe for the patient's skin type is paramount, as the risk of epidermal injury is greater in higher Fitzpatrick skin phototypes (SPT).[26] Given that epidermal melanin acts as a competing chromophore in individuals with higher SPT, longer-wavelength lasers such as the diode (800–810 nm) and neodymium:yttrium aluminum garnet (Nd:YAG 1064 nm) lasers are preferred for men of African ancestry with high SPT. The 1064-nm Nd:YAG laser has the safest profile for this patient population and therefore is strongly preferred.[26] Combining topical eflornithine hydrochloride 13.9% cream (to slow down hair growth) along with long-pulsed 1064-nm Nd:YAG laser hair removal has been shown to be more effective than laser hair removal alone.[27]

FOLLICULITIS KELOIDALIS NUCHAE
Epidemiology

FKN, also known as acne keloidalis nuchae, is a follicular disorder primarily seen in men of African ancestry with Afro-textured hair. However, it may rarely also be seen in women; the ratio of affected men to affected women is 20:1.[28,29] In an epidemiologic study by Khumalo and colleagues,[30] FKN was diagnosed in 4.7% of South African boys in the last year of school, in 10.5% of adult men, and 0.3% of adult women. In a study by Adegbidi and colleagues,[31] FKN accounted for 0.7% of all dermatology consultations at a university hospital in Benin, while Salami and colleagues[32] reported a prevalence of 9.4% of dermatology consultations at a Nigerian university hospital. FKN occurs in 0.5% of African Americans.[33] Men often attribute the beginning of FKN to an infection from unclean barber instruments,[34] although this has not been substantiated in published studies. Khumalo and colleagues[30] reported an association between FKN and bleeding from haircuts. The papules of FKN may be injured during the hair-cutting process because of the force required to perform haircuts on patients with tightly coiled hair texture.[35] In the setting of shared, unsterilized hair clippers, transmission of human immunodeficiency virus and other blood-borne diseases are a risk.[35]

Pathogenesis

The etiology of FKN remains incompletely understood.[36] FKN usually occurs in men with frequent and close haircuts.[37] It may also occur in women who shape the hair of the posterior neck with a razor.[34] Shapero and Shapero[38] hypothesized that FKN is initiated by a mechanically induced folliculitis that becomes extensive enough to result in scar formation. Based on a histopathologic study, Sperling and colleagues[39] argue that FKN is a primary cicatricial alopecia that is not causally associated with ingrown hairs or bacterial infection.

Reported contributory factors to FKN include trauma, chronic irritation, seborrhea, infection, and elevated testosterone levels.[34,40] Sources of mechanical irritation that may exacerbate or potentially contribute to the development FKN include friction from high-collared shirts, sports helmets, and other garments or equipment.[34,38] George and colleagues[40] found that 58% of Nigerian patients with FKN reported using a uniquely shaped comb, called an Afro wooden or plastic comb, frequently referred to as an Afro pick in the United States. The investigators pointed out that while using this comb, users often mechanically scrape the surface of the scalp.[40]

The development of FKN in a black man following an episode of zoster on the scalp has been reported.[41] Keloidal plaques in patients with FKN may not develop on any other part of the body except for the occipital scalp. FKN patients, unlike patients with multiple keloids on the body, often do not have a personal or family history of keloids.[34] Understanding why keloidal plaques are site restricted in FKN may provide clues to the pathogenesis of FKN and keloids.

The histology of FKN usually consists of chronic perifollicular inflammation and destruction of hair follicles.[38] Features of transepithelial hair elimination similar to those found in perforating disorders, including granuloma annulare, reactive perforating collagenosis, elastosis perforans serpiginosa, and chondrodermatitis nodularis chronica helicis, have also been described.[42] In a study of Nigerian patients by George and colleagues,[40] the nape of the neck/occipital scalp was found to have an increased (almost double) number of mast cells compared with the anterior scalp. Moreover, dermal capillary dilation was more profound on the nape of the neck.[40] The large number of mast cells in this location may contribute to a pruritic sensation prompting rubbing and manipulation of the skin.[38] Genetic predisposition may also influence the density of mast cells in the scalp.[38]

Clinical Features

FKN is characterized by fibrotic papules on the occipital scalp, typically involving the nape of the neck (**Fig. 6**). Pustules and/or crusted papules can also be observed, especially when secondary infection occurs (**Fig. 7**). Severe secondary infections can result in abscess formation. Pruritus is common, and patients frequently admit to scratching or rubbing the affected areas. In severe or long-standing cases the papules may coalesce into a large, hairless fibrotic plaques or nodules. Tufted hairs (multiple hair shafts emerging from a single follicular opening) may also be present.[1,30] FKN can be disfiguring and may adversely affect self-esteem.

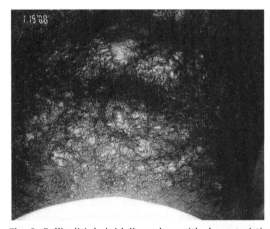

Fig. 6. Folliculitis keloidalis nuchae with characteristic involvement of the posterior scalp and nape of neck.

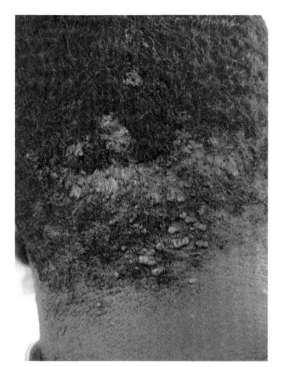

Fig. 7. Folliculitis keloidalis nuchae with secondary infection. Note crusted papules on the occipital scalp.

Management

The first step in the management of FKN is initiating preventive measures to minimize disease progression or exacerbation. Such measures include avoidance of mechanical irritation from shirt collars, hats, short haircuts, and self-manipulation; and the use of topical antimicrobial cleansers (eg, chlorhexidine or povidone iodine) to prevent secondary infection.

Mild to moderate cases of FKN can be improved with the use of potent and ultrapotent topical corticosteroids. Topical therapies are generally sufficient when the papules are 3 mm or smaller and no nodules are present. To prevent atrophy and other side effects of corticosteroids, an alternating 2-week cycle (ie, 2 weeks on, 2 weeks off) of the steroid is a useful approach. In a study by Callender and colleagues,[43] alternate 2-week cycles of clobetasol propionate 0.05% foam twice daily for 8 weeks (followed by 4 weeks of betamethasone valerate 0.12% foam twice daily if lesions persisted) demonstrated significant decreases in papule/pustule counts at week 12. Topical clindamycin gel or foam can also be used in conjunction with topical corticosteroids, especially when pustules are present. For larger papules and plaques, 20 to 40 mg/mL triamcinolone acetonide intralesionally should be added to the regimen. Oral doxycycline or minocycline are useful for extensive cases because of their anti-inflammatory and anti-microbial effects (in cases of secondary infection).

Surgical excision can be considered for severe cases of FKN that are resistant to medical therapy, especially when large (eg, ≥3 cm) fibrotic plaques or nodules are present. Recommended techniques for surgical management of FKN include excising a horizontal ellipse that involves the posterior hairline and extends to the subcutaneous fat, followed by either second-intention healing[44,45] or primary closure.[46] Excision by carbon dioxide laser[47] and electrosurgery[45] (followed by second-intention healing) have also been reported. Published studies with long-term follow-up are currently lacking and, therefore, there is a paucity of data on recurrence rates from surgical excision of FKN. Notwithstanding this limitation, the rates of recurrence after excision of FKN appear to be low, in contrast to those associated with keloid excisions.

Laser hair removal can be considered as an alternative or adjunct to conventional therapies.[48,49] In a study of 16 patients with FKN who underwent 5 sessions of laser hair removal with the long-pulsed Nd:YAG laser, significant reductions in papule count, plaque count, and plaque size were observed.[49]

SUMMARY

PFB and FKN are potentially disfiguring follicular disorders that are primarily seen in men of African ancestry who have Afro-textured hair. Recent advances have brought prevention strategies and effective treatment within reach for most patients. Modification of grooming practices in combination with the appropriate use of both pharmacologic and procedural interventions is generally effective in controlling these diseases. Notwithstanding recent advances, PFB and FKN remain therapeutically challenging, relapses are common, and potential barriers to care exist (eg, limited access to laser hair removal, the need for frequent office visits, and considerable costs of treatment). Further research is warranted to better elucidate the mechanisms of disease, optimize treatment outcomes, and, ultimately, improve the quality of life of patients with these disorders.

REFERENCES

1. Coley MK, Kelly AP, Alexis AF. Pseudofolliculitis barbae and acne keloidalis nuchae. In: Alexis AF, Barbosa VH, editors. Skin of color a practical guide to dermatologic diagnosis and treatment. 1st edition. New York: Springer; 2013. p. 123–38.

2. Quarles FN, Coley MK, Alexis AF. Dermatological disorders in men of African descent. In: Dadzie OE, Petit A, Alexis AF, editors. Ethnic dermatology principles and practice. 1st edition. Chichester, West Sussex: Wiley-Blackwell; 2013. p. 241–56.

3. Coley MK, Alexis AF. Dermatologic conditions in men of African ancestry. Expert Rev Dermatol 2009;4:595–609.

4. Perry PK, Cook-Bolden FE, Rahman Z, et al. Defining pseudofolliculitis barbae in 2001: a review of the literature and current trends. J Am Acad Dermatol 2002;46(2 Suppl Understanding):S113–9.

5. Alexander AM, Delph WI. Pseudofolliculitis barbae in the military. A medical, administrative and social problem. J Natl Med Assoc 1974;66(6):459–64, 479.

6. Edlich RF, Haines PC, Nichter LS, et al. Pseudofolliculitis barbae with keloids. J Emerg Med 1986;4(4):283–6.

7. Bridgeman-Shah S. The medical and surgical therapy of pseudofolliculitis barbae. Dermatol Ther 2004;17(2):158–63.

8. Kelly AP. Pseudofolliculitis barbae. In: Kelly AP, Taylor SC, editors. Dermatology for skin of color. New York: McGraw-Hill; 2009. p. 211–6.

9. Brown LA Jr. Pathogenesis and treatment of pseudofolliculitis barbae. Cutis 1983;32(4):373–5.

10. Halder RM. Pseudofolliculitis barbae and related disorders. Dermatol Clin 1988;6(3):407–12.

11. Winter H, Schissel D, Parry DA, et al. An unusual Ala12Thr polymorphism in the 1A alpha-helical segment of the companion layer-specific keratin K6hf: evidence for a risk factor in the etiology of the common hair disorder pseudofolliculitis barbae. J Invest Dermatol 2004;122(3):652–7.

12. Kelly AP. Pseudofolliculitis barbae. In: Arndt K, LeBoit P, Robinson J, et al, editors. Cutaneous medicine and surgery. vol. 1. 1996. Philadelphia: W.B. Saunders p. 499–503.

13. Brauner GJ, Flandermeyer KL. Pseudofolliculitis barbae. Medical consequences of interracial friction in the US Army. Cutis 1979;23(1):61–6.

14. McMichael AJ. Hair and scalp disorders in ethnic populations. Dermatol Clin 2003;21(4):629–44.

15. Cowley K, Vanoosthuyze K. Insights into shaving and its impact on skin. Br J Dermatol 2012;166(Suppl 1):6–12.

16. Daniel A, Gustafson CJ, Zupkosky PJ, et al. Shave frequency and regimen variation effects on the management of pseudofolliculitis barbae. J Drugs Dermatol 2013;12(4):410–8.

17. Alexander AM. Evaluation of a foil-guarded shaver in the management of pseudofolliculitis barbae. Cutis 1981;27(5):534–7, 540–32.

18. Kindred C, Oresajo CO, Yatskayer M, et al. Comparative evaluation of men's depilatory composition versus razor in black men. Cutis 2011;88(2):98–103.

19. Cook-Bolden FE, Barba A, Halder R, et al. Twice-daily applications of benzoyl peroxide 5%/clindamycin 1% gel versus vehicle in the treatment of pseudofolliculitis barbae. Cutis 2004;73(Suppl 6):18–24.

20. Kligman AM, Mills OH Jr. Pseudofolliculitis of the beard and topically applied tretinoin. Arch Dermatol 1973;107(4):551–2.

21. Coley MK, Alexis AF. Managing common dermatoses in skin of color. Semin Cutan Med Surg 2009;28(2):63–70.

22. Bulengo-Ransby SM, Griffiths CE, Kimbrough-Green CK, et al. Topical tretinoin (retinoic acid) therapy for hyperpigmented lesions caused by inflammation of the skin in black patients. N Engl J Med 1993;328(20):1438–43.

23. Weaver SM 3rd, Sagaral EC. Treatment of pseudofolliculitis barbae using the long-pulse Nd:YAG laser on skin types V and VI. Dermatol Surg 2003;29(12):1187–91.

24. Smith EP, Winstanley D, Ross EV. Modified super-long pulse 810 nm diode laser in the treatment of pseudofolliculitis barbae in skin types V and VI. Dermatol Surg 2005;31(3):297–301.

25. Ross EV, Cooke LM, Timko AL, et al. Treatment of pseudofolliculitis barbae in skin types IV, V, and VI with a long-pulsed neodymium:yttrium aluminum garnet laser. J Am Acad Dermatol 2002;47(2):263–70.

26. Alexis AF. Lasers and light-based therapies in ethnic skin: treatment options and recommendations for Fitzpatrick skin types V and VI. Br J Dermatol 2013;169(S3):91–7.

27. Xia Y, Cho S, Howard RS, et al. Topical eflornithine hydrochloride improves the effectiveness of standard laser hair removal for treating pseudofolliculitis barbae: a randomized, double-blinded, placebo-controlled trial. J Am Acad Dermatol 2012;67(4):694–9.

28. Kelly AP. Pseudofolliculitis barbae and acne keloidalis nuchae. Dermatol Clin 2003;21(4):645–53.

29. Dinehart SM, Tanner L, Mallory SB, et al. Acne keloidalis in women. Cutis 1989;44(3):250–2.

30. Dadzie OE, Petit A, Alexis AF. Ethnic dermatology: principles and practice. Chichester (West Sussex): Wiley-Blackwell; 2013.

31. Adegbidi H, Atadokpede F, do Ango-Padonou F, et al. Keloid acne of the neck: epidemiological studies over 10 years. Int J Dermatol 2005;44(Suppl 1):49–50.

32. Salami T, Omeife H, Samuel S. Prevalence of acne keloidalis nuchae in Nigerians. Int J Dermatol 2007;46(5):482–4.

33. Ogunbiyi A, George A. Acne keloidalis in females: case report and review of literature. J Natl Med Assoc 2005;97(5):736–8.

34. Khumalo NP, Gumedze F, Lehloenya R. Folliculitis keloidalis nuchae is associated with the risk for bleeding from haircuts. Int J Dermatol 2011;50(10):1212–6.

35. Khumalo NP. Folliculitis keloidalis nuchae, bleeding from haircuts, and potential HIV transmission. Int J Dermatol 2012;51(Suppl 1):21–3, 24–6.

36. Rodney IJ, Onwudiwe OC, Callender VD, et al. Hair and scalp disorders in ethnic populations. J Drugs Dermatol 2013;12(4):420–7.

37. Khumalo NP, Jessop S, Gumedze F, et al. Hairdressing is associated with scalp disease in African schoolchildren. Br J Dermatol 2007;157(1):106–10.

38. Shapero J, Shapero H. Acne keloidalis nuchae is scar and keloid formation secondary to mechanically induced folliculitis. J Cutan Med Surg 2011;15(4):238–40.

39. Sperling LC, Homoky C, Pratt L, et al. Acne keloidalis is a form of primary scarring alopecia. Arch Dermatol 2000;136(4):479–84.

40. George AO, Akanji AO, Nduka EU, et al. Clinical, biochemical and morphologic features of acne keloidalis in a black population. Int J Dermatol 1993; 32(10):714–6.

41. Bellavista S, D'Antuono A, Gaspari V, et al. Acne keloidalis nuchae on herpes zoster scar in an HIV patient: isotopic response or not? G Ital Dermatol Venereol 2012;147(2):223–6.

42. Goette DK, Berger TG. Acne keloidalis nuchae. A transepithelial elimination disorder. Int J Dermatol 1987;26(7):442–4.

43. Callender VD, Young CM, Haverstock CL, et al. An open label study of clobetasol propionate 0.05% and betamethasone valerate 0.12% foams in the treatment of mild to moderate acne keloidalis. Cutis 2005;75(6):317–21.

44. Glenn MJ, Bennett RG, Kelly AP. Acne keloidalis nuchae: treatment with excision and second-intention healing. J Am Acad Dermatol 1995;33 (2 Pt 1):243–6.

45. Beckett N, Lawson C, Cohen G. Electrosurgical excision of acne keloidalis nuchae with secondary intention healing. J Clin Aesthet Dermatol 2011; 4(1):36–9.

46. Gloster HM Jr. The surgical management of extensive cases of acne keloidalis nuchae. Arch Dermatol 2000;136(11):1376–9.

47. Kantor GR, Ratz JL, Wheeland RG. Treatment of acne keloidalis nuchae with carbon dioxide laser. J Am Acad Dermatol 1986;14(2 Pt 1):263–7.

48. Shah GK. Efficacy of diode laser for treating acne keloidalis nuchae. Indian J Dermatol Venereol Leprol 2005;71(1):31–4.

49. Esmat SM, Abdel Hay RM, Abu Zeid OM, et al. The efficacy of laser-assisted hair removal in the treatment of acne keloidalis nuchae; a pilot study. Eur J Dermatol 2012;22(5):645–50.

New Insights on Keloids, Hypertrophic Scars, and Striae

Sara Ud-Din, MSc[a,b], Ardeshir Bayat, MBBS, MRCS, PhD[a,b,*]

KEYWORDS

- Keloid disease • Hypertrophic scars • Striae distensae • Assessment • Treatment • Prevention
- Focused treatment options

KEY POINTS

- Management of hypertrophic scars, keloid disease, and striae distensae in dark pigmented skin remains a clinical challenge.
- There are various treatment modalities; however, there is no single therapy that is advocated for hypertrophic scars, keloid disease, or striae distensae.
- Clinical risk scoring of abnormal scarring and striae distensae may allow those with high risk to be offered prophylactic therapies and preventive measures in advance.
- A focused history involving patient's symptoms, signs, and quality of life/psychosocial well-being should be used in order to define goals and direct treatment options.
- Regular follow-up should be undertaken in order to assess whether treatment is effective, needs continuation for prevention of recurrence, or should be stopped.

INTRODUCTION

Cutaneous dermal injury inevitably leads to scar formation.[1] The reparative process involves inflammation, granulation tissue formation, and matrix remodeling, which can result in varying degrees of dermal fibrosis (**Fig. 1**).[1] In certain individuals and anatomic sites, excessive fibrosis may lead to hypertrophic scar or keloid disease (KD) formation (**Fig. 2**).[2] In contrast, endogenous factors including mechanical stretching and hormonal influences can lead to dermal dehiscence, which can result in the development of striae distensae (SD) (see **Fig. 2**).[3]

Keloid scars are raised reticular dermal lesions that spread beyond the confines of the original wound and invade the surrounding healthy skin (**Table 1**).[4] They can develop up to, or even beyond, 1 year after the injury and do not tend to regress spontaneously.[4] Scars are erythematous, raised, firm areas of fibrotic skin that are limited to the original wound site.[5] Hypertrophic scars (HTS) tend to form within the first month after the injury but can become flatter and more pliable

Funding Sources: Nil.

Conflict of Interest: Nil.

[a] Plastic and Reconstructive Surgery Research, Manchester Institute of Biotechnology, University of Manchester, 131 Princess Street, Manchester M1 7DN, UK; [b] Plastic and Reconstructive Surgery Research, Faculty of Medical and Human Sciences, Institute of Inflammation and Repair, University Hospital of South Manchester NHS Foundation Trust, Manchester Academic Health Science Centre, University of Manchester, Manchester, UK

* Corresponding author. Plastic and Reconstructive Surgery Research, Manchester Institute of Biotechnology, University of Manchester, 131 Princess Street, Manchester M1 7DN, UK.

E-mail address: ardeshir.bayat@manchester.ac.uk

Dermatol Clin 32 (2014) 193–209

http://dx.doi.org/10.1016/j.det.2013.11.002

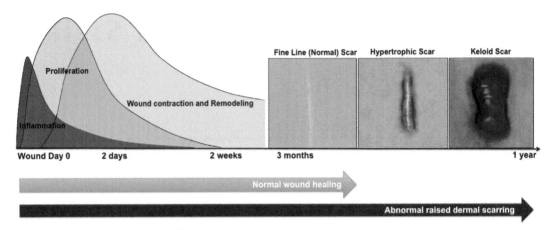

Fig. 1. The spectrum of wound healing.

over time and often resolve within a year.[6] Both KD and HTS tend to be pruritic and painful and can be cosmetically unsightly.[6] Their prevalence ranges from 4.5% to 16% of the population and they are thought to be most common in individuals with dark pigmented skin.[7] KD and HTS are considered to be an important clinical problem in certain ethnic populations, because there is a higher prevalence in individuals with dark pigmented skin.[8–10] KD, in particular, is reported to be especially high in individuals of African, Asian, and Hispanic descent.[11]

SD are linear bands of atrophic skin that occur following excessive dermal stretching (see **Table 1**).[12] Most SD have been reported in pregnant women and adolescents and in long-term steroid use (**Fig. 3**).[13,14] SD often exhibit scarlike features because early striae (striae rubrae) appear erythematous and late striae (striae albae) show hypopigmentation and dermal fibrosis.[15] There are also 2 additional types of SD: striae nigrae and striae caerulea, which occur in people with dark skin because of increased melanization.[16] Striae nigrae appear as black bands of atrophic skin, whereas striae caerulea have a blue appearance.[16] SD severity has been noted to be more severe in black African women compared with white people within the same geographic region.[17,18]

Many different treatment modalities exist that claim to improve HTS, KD, and SD. Nevertheless, these lesions are difficult to eradicate using commonly available treatments.[2,6,11] There is no single therapy that can effectively eradicate abnormal skin scars and SD. No single treatment plan has been advocated for both scars and SD, and the literature provides no gold standard therapy, which is hampered by a paucity of level 1 evidence. Therefore, this article summarizes a management strategy and provides an overview of the most current and available treatment options for managing KD, HTS, and SD in patients with dark pigmented skin.

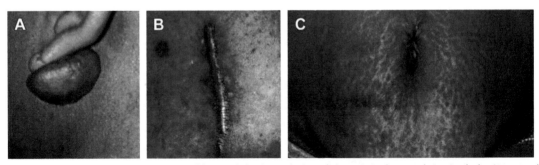

Fig. 2. (A) Earlobe keloid scarring spread beyond the boundaries of the original wound site in dark pigmented skin. (B) A hypertrophic scar remaining within the boundaries of the original wound in a dark-skinned individual. (C) Striae distensae (SD) following pregnancy on the abdomen with dark pigmented skin.

Table 1
The characteristics of keloid scars, hypertrophic scars and SD

	Hypertrophic Scars	Keloid Scars	Striae Distensae (Striae Rubrae)	Striae Distensae (Striae Albae)
Onset	Develop soon after injury	Can develop months after injury	Usually occur during pregnancy, adolescence and obesity	Usually occur during pregnancy, adolescence and obesity
Physical characteristics	Remain within the confines of the wound	Spread beyond the boundaries of the wound	Early stage striae, raised red linear lesions	Pale, depressed and finely wrinkled lesions
Recurrence	Reduced risk of recurrence following treatment including surgery	High risk of recurrence following treatment including surgery	No risk of recurrence, although difficult to treat	No risk of recurrence, although difficult to treat
Occurrence	Usually located in high tension areas	Usually occur in areas including the earlobes and high tension areas such as the sternum	Common locations include the abdomen, breasts, thighs, hips	Common locations include the abdomen, breasts, thighs, hips
Skin Type	Associations with fair skin types	High association in dark pigmented skin	Due to mechanical stretching of the skin and hormonal imbalance. Skin type can affect treatment choice	Due to mechanical stretching of the skin and hormonal imbalance. Skin type can affect treatment choice
Permanent	Can regress spontaneously	Do not regress	Temporary form of striae	Permanent form of striae
Histological characteristics	Increased fibroblast density	Increased fibroblast density and proliferation rates	Thin epidermis, fine collagen bundles arranged in straight parallel lines	Thin epidermis, fine collagen bundles arranged in straight parallel lines

PATIENT EVALUATION OVERVIEW

A thorough clinical assessment should be performed in order to tailor the appropriate management strategy to an individual affected with abnormal scarring or SD. This assessment should include a full medical history of the individual; any family history of KD, HTS, or SD; and presence of any psychosocial issues. In addition, the assessment should include a detailed history of the scar or striae, noting the size, contour, location, pliability, color, and any associated symptoms such as pruritus and pain. Furthermore, it is essential to take digital photographs before and after treatments to monitor any physical changes.

A range of instruments exist to monitor and quantify the physical and physiologic characteristics of KD and HTS by objective measures. Devices are used to measure the color of a scar such as spectrophotometric intracutaneous analysis, which provides a pigmentary status of the first 2 mm of the skin through reflectance and absorption of light.[19] This device provides quantitative measurements of hemoglobin, melanin, and collagen levels. Epiluminescence colorimetry has also been used to identify the color of SD.[16] Because this technique provides visualization of melanin, this may help in the visualization of SD in darker skin types.[20]

Furthermore, full-field laser perfusion imaging provides quantitative measurements of vascularity that can evaluate the blood flow at the scar site.[21] Scar volume is an important characteristic when assessing a lesion. Three-dimensional imaging devices are available for analyzing the volume, planimetry, and texture of skin scars and SD.[22,23] Furthermore, ultrasonography techniques, such as the tissue ultrasound palpation system and DermaScan systems, can be used to quantify the total depth of a scar.[24] Tools such as the tissue tonometer have been shown to be useful in assessing

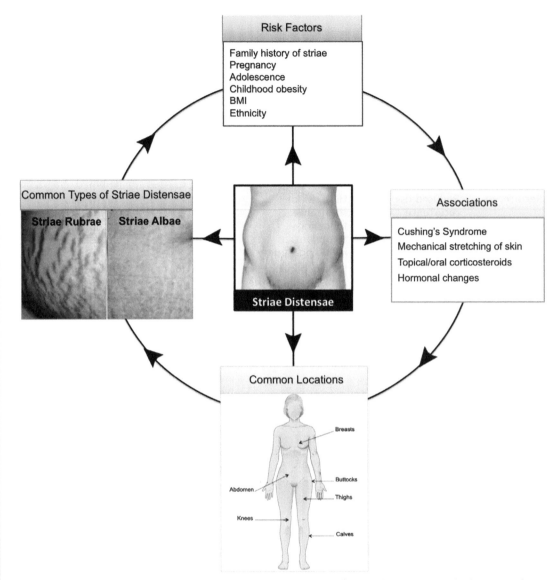

Fig. 3. The risk factors, associations, common locations, and types of striae distensae. BMI, body mass index.

skin scar pliability.[25] Techniques such as optical coherence tomography (OCT) have recently been used in assessing KD and HTS to visualize skin morphology and measure dimensions in the skin layers.[26] In addition, in vivo confocal microscopy has been used in assessing KD, HTS, and SD by performing optical horizontal sectioning within human tissue, allowing a view of sections of the skin.[27,28]

Because each patient is unique, it is important to create a tailored treatment protocol guided by evidence observed in effective therapies, remembering always to address the patient's individual needs. A direct approach incorporating the patient's symptoms, signs, quality of life, and well-being should be of paramount importance in order to target treatment effectively. In addition, regular follow-up is essential to ensure that treatment is effective, to identify any side effects, and to cease treatment in cases with successful outcomes.

MANAGEMENT GOALS

It is important to treat the patient's clinical problems by first addressing the presenting complaints. A focused approach in targeting the individual's symptoms, such as pain, pruritus, and inflammation, should take priority before aiming to reduce the lesion (in the case of keloid and HTS). Most of the therapeutic approaches are used indiscriminately for management of both HTS and keloids. However, clinical differentiation between HTS and keloid scars is vital before the initiation of any treatment, because of increased recurrence rates with keloids. For SD, goals of therapy are to provide long-lasting improvements in both pigmentation and texture of striae, with minimal side effects. Furthermore, it is important to evaluate the patients continuously following each treatment intervention, record progress and compare with the condition using a digital photograph, assess for side effects, evaluate objectively treatment, prevent complications, and cease therapy when indicated.

PHARMACOLOGIC TREATMENT OPTIONS

There are various pharmacologic treatment options that are available to treat KD, HTS, and SD. The most current and commonly used treatments are discussed later (**Table 2**).

Intralesional Injections

Intralesional injections of corticosteroids are considered, by the International Clinical Recommendations on Scar Management, the standard first-line treatment of KD and a secondary treatment of HTS.[29–31] There are several corticosteroids used for raised dermal scarring in dark pigmented skin, such as dexamethasone, hydrocortisone acetate, and methyl prednisolone, and the most common type of injection is triamcinolone acetonide.[32] Injection of corticosteroids leads to the regression of KD and HTS by reducing the

inflammatory process, altering collagen gene expression, and inhibiting collagen and glycosaminoglycan synthesis.[33,34] The effectiveness of single or multiple injections can be variable and recurrence rates range from 9% to 50%.[9,35] Triamcinolone acetonide can be used in a combination of doses (1–40 mg/mL).[29,36–39] Three to 4 injections of triamcinolone acetonide (10–40 mg/mL) every 3 to 4 weeks are generally sufficient, although occasionally injections continue for 6 months or more.[37,40] A recent case series conducted by our team evaluated the response rate of triamcinolone acetonide injections in 65 patients with KD including patients with dark pigmented skin.[41] Triamcinolone acetonide was injected at a concentration of 10 mg/1 mL. The dose was 2 to 3 mg, with a maximum of 5 mg at any one site. A total dose of 30 mg was administered in line with British National Formulary (BNF) guidelines. The results showed that there was a 77% positive response rate, which was defined by an improvement in signs (color, height, contour) and symptoms (pain, pruritus) associated with raised dermal skin scarring. This finding shows level 4 evidence (level of evidence [LOE]-4) of the positive effects of triamcinolone acetonide for the treatment of KD and in patients with dark pigmented skin.

Berman and colleagues[36] conducted a randomized controlled study (LOE-1) involving 20 patients of varying skin types, comparing intralesional steroid with etanercept in KD.[36] Triamcinolone acetonide improved 11 out of 12 parameters assessed compared with etanercept, which improved 5 out of 12. The investigators reported that scar evaluations were blinded; however, it is unclear how this was achieved, because assessments were completed by the same investigator.

Table 2
The pharmacologic treatment options for the management of keloid scars, hypertrophic scars, and SD

Treatment	Indication	Dosage	Duration	Side Effects
Corticosteroids	KD + HTS	1–40 mg/mL	Maximum dosage of 3 injections every 3–4 wk	Telangiectasia, atrophy, hypopigmentation, pain
5-Fluorouracil	KD + HTS	50 mg/mL	Weekly doses. Variable duration depending on response	Ulceration, hyperpigmentation, pain
Tretinoin	SD	0.025%–0.1%	Daily application with variable duration depending on response	Mild skin irritation
Glycolic acid	SD	10%–35%	1–2 min repeated monthly for up to 6 mo	Stronger concentrations can lead to irreversible scar formation

Darzi[39] conducted a randomized controlled trial (RCT) (LOE-1) and compared 100 scars (KD and HTS) in 65 patients. Each received either beta radiation alone, or in combination with surgery, or triamcinolone acetonide. They showed that the scar symptoms improved (72%) and flattening of the scars were noted (64%) after receiving this therapy.[39] This treatment can be painful and associated side effects include telangiectasia, atrophy, and pigmentary changes (**Fig. 4**). Hypopigmentation often continues for years after treatment and is more highly visible in dark pigmented skin.[6,40]

5-Fluorouracil (5-FU) is a pyrimidine analogue that is converted to a substrate that causes the inhibition of DNA synthesis.[42] 5-FU is administered via intralesional injection either in single or multiple doses or at the time of surgery, and it is thought to reduce scarring by suppressing fibroblast proliferation.[43,44] It has been advocated that intralesional injections of 5-FU should be administered once weekly at doses of 50 mg/mL for approximately 7 sessions.[45] A comparative study (LOE-2) of 5 patients comparing various treatment regimes of 5-FU showed that the therapy was effective for HTS, as well as KD.[44] Scars that were inflamed, firm, and symptomatic responded more significantly to 5-FU monotherapy or polytherapy.

A prospective study (LOE-4) conducted in India investigated the use of intralesional 5-FU and surgical excision in 28 patients, some with dark pigmented skin and with earlobe keloid scars.[46] 5-FU was a useful method of reducing the recurrence of KD, because 27 of the patients required no further treatment in 22 months.

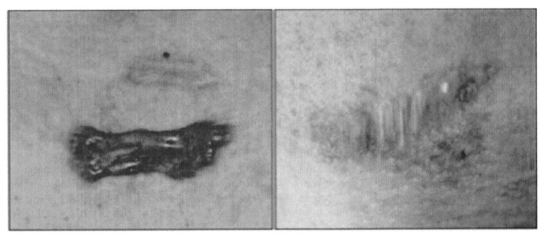

Telangiectasias   **Steroid deposit**

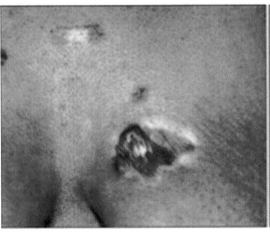
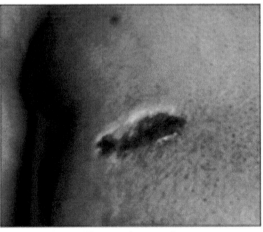

Areas of hypopigmentation   **Dermal atrophy**

Fig. 4. The side effects of telangiectasias and steroid deposit following corticosteroid injection treatment. In addition, hypopigmentation and dermal atrophy are shown following corticosteroid injections in dark pigmented skin.

A double-blind RCT (LOE-1) recently tested the effects of 5-FU and topical silicone in 50 patients who were split into 2 groups, 1 treatment and 1 control group.[47] The sample group included patients with dark pigmented skin as well as white people. The treated group had less recurrence (4% treated, compared with 22% control) and a greater number of patients who were keloid free (75% treated, compared with 43% control) compared with the control group. Furthermore, Sadeghinia and Sadheginia[48] compared 5-FU with intralesional steroid injections in 40 patients with KD. This double-blind RCT showed that the 5-FU group had significantly better results in the treatment of KD than the intralesional steroid group. There can be significant side effects, such as ulceration, and pain.[45,49,50] Hyperpigmentation can also occur, although this has been reported to improve after discontinuation of treatment.[51]

Tretinoin

Tretinoin is a vitamin A–derived, nonpeptidic, small lipophilic molecule and has been used in the treatment of SD.[15,52,53] This molecule works by inducing collagen synthesis and encouraging fibroblast activity.[53] Dosage and duration of tretinoin cream varies in the literature, but the common doses used are 0.1%, 0.05%, or 0.025%, and it has been advocated this should be applied daily.[54] There have been positive responses using this topical agent in striae rubrae and poor responses noted in striae albae.[54,55] Mild irritation has been the most common side effect noted but this ceases when treatment ends.[56] A double-blind, placebo controlled study (LOE-1) investigated the response of pregnancy-related abdominal striae to tretinoin cream (0.025%) applied for 7 months in 11 patients of varying ethnicities, including in dark pigmented skin.[57] However, no differences were noted between the groups and no improvement in the SD in the treated group compared with the placebo group. The small sample size in this study may have contributed to these results.

A double-blind RCT (LOE-1) investigated the efficacy of topical tretinoin 0.1% compared with a vehicle cream on 26 white patients with SD.[52] At 24 weeks, 80% of patients in the tretinoin group had an improvement in their SD compared with the vehicle group (8%). However, it is possible that these results should not be generalized to the population because only white patients were included, therefore this treatment may not be as effective for dark pigmented skin. Further trials are necessary in order to determine the effects of tretinoin on dark pigmented skin.

Acid Peels

Acid peel treatments are used to improve and smooth the texture of the skin using a chemical solution that causes the skin peel to stimulate dermal fibroblasts and enhance collagen synthesis.[56–58] A concentration of 10% to 35% has been advocated as the optimal level because concentrations stronger than this can cause irreversible scar formation.[59] In addition, hyperpigmentation can be a side effect following this treatment.[58] Treatment can be applied for 1 to 2 minutes at each application and repeated monthly for up to 6 months.[60] Glycolic acid has been used to enhance collagen synthesis.[57] An increased epidermal thickness, elastin content, and reduced SD width following the use of glycolic acid has also been noted.[57] Furthermore, a more recent double-blind controlled study (LOE-2) by Mazzarello and colleagues[60] investigated the effect of glycolic acid on 40 patients of mixed ethnicities with SD. Striae rubrae were decreased in SD width and hemoglobin levels. Striae albae also showed an increase in melanin levels. However, there is no report of randomization or blinding, and explanation of how patients were allocated to each group is lacking. There is limited evidence for the effect of acid peels on SD, especially in dark pigmented skin.

NONPHARMACOLOGIC TREATMENT OPTIONS

There are various nonpharmacologic treatment options that are available to treat KD, HTS, and SD. The most current and commonly used treatments are discussed here (Table 3).

Silicone Gel

Silicone gel is a medical-grade silicone and has been used in the management of HTS and KD.[29,61] There are various forms of topical silicone such as liquid,[62] gel cushion,[63] creams,[64] spray,[65] and vitamin-supplemented silicone,[66] with the most common being silicone gel sheeting.[29] Silicone gel sheeting is a soft dressing made from dimethylsiloxane cross-linked polymer.[67] Silicone gel sheeting is used regularly as monotherapy in raised dermal scarring to maintain skin hydration.[68,69] It should be worn for between 10 and 24 hours a day.[70,71] A small number of side effects have been reported, such as pruritus, rash, and skin breakdown.[72,73] However, investigators have shown that these problems resolve quickly if patients keep the area clean and if patient compliance is ensured using education.[74,75]

de Oliveira and colleagues[74] conducted an RCT (LOE-1) on 26 patients with HTS and keloid scars

Table 3
The treatment options for the management of keloid scars, hypertrophic scars, and striae distensae

Treatment	Type of Lesion	Application	Duration	Side Effects
Silicone gel	KD + HTS	Sheet dressing	12–24 h a day	Pruritus, rash, skin breakdown
Cryotherapy	KD + HTS	Thaw cycles of 20–30 s, 1–12 times	3–4 wk, between 3–6 treatments	Permanent hypopigmentation and hyperpigmentation, blistering, pain
Photodynamic therapy	KD	3–5 treatments	Weekly sessions	Short-term pain and inflammation, long-term hypopigmentation/hyperpigmentation
UVA/UVB	SD	10 sessions	Weekly sessions	Erythema
Electrical stimulation	KD + HTS	Fenzian device: 30-min sessions	Regular daily sessions until symptoms cease	Inflammation in early stage of treatment
Lasers	SD, KD, HTS	1–24 treatments	Intervals of 4–8 wk	Hypopigmentation, pain, pruritus, purpuric spots

Abbreviations: UVA, ultraviolet A; UVB, ultraviolet B.

and compared silicone gel sheeting with a dressing and an untreated control group.[74] There was no significant difference noted between the treatment groups. The international guidelines on scar management published in 2002 promote silicone gel sheeting as first-line therapy for linear HTS, widespread burn HTS, and minor KD.[29] However, a Cochrane Review in 2013, determining the effectiveness of silicone gel sheeting in the treatment and prevention of keloid and hypertrophic scarring, concluded that there is weak evidence for silicone gel sheeting improving abnormal scarring in high-risk individuals, that studies are of poor quality, and thus that the efficacy of silicone gel sheets remains unclear.[76]

Cryotherapy

Cryotherapy is a low-temperature treatment that is used to freeze skin lesions.[77] Cryotherapy is thought to induce vascular damage that may lead to anoxia and ultimately tissue necrosis when used for the treatment of KD and HTS.[77] Repeated cyotherapy sessions have been suggested to have a beneficial effect on the outcome of HTS and KD and prevent recurrences.[78,79] The scar should have thaw cycles of 20 to 30 seconds, and this should be repeated 1 to 12 times in total, depending on the size of the scar.[80,81] It has been advocated that treatments should be performed every 3 to 4 weeks with between 3 and 6 treatments often needed. Common side effects include permanent hypopigmentation and hyperpigmentation, blistering, delayed healing, and

postoperative pain.[77,82,83] There is a lack of evidence pertaining to individuals with dark pigmented skin.

A double blind RCT (LOE-1) compared cryotherapy with intralesional steroid injections and untreated controls in 11 patients with acne keloid scars.[81] Cryotherapy was more effective (85%) than intralesional steroid injections. In addition, a comparative study (LOE-2) showed significant improvements using cryotherapy combined with intralesional corticosteroid, versus cryotherapy or intralesional corticosteroid alone, in 10 patients with KD.[77] However, the blinding technique was not described and the ethnicity of the patients was not clear.

Topical Oils/Creams

There are various topical treatments available for managing SD.[84–86] They are predominantly used as a prophylactic in order to prevent SD from developing during pregnancy.[87] A Cochrane Review in 2012 evaluated 6 topical agents in more than 800 women with SD.[88] The studies used had small sample sizes and there was a lack of statistically significant evidence to support the use in treating SD.

A double-blind controlled study (LOE-2) conducted by our team evaluated the use of topical silicone gel and a placebo gel on 20 women with abdominal SD.[89] The participants were of various ethnicities from skin types I to V. Gels were applied daily for 6 weeks to each side of the abdomen. Melanin increased, and vascularity, collagen, elastin, and pliability decreased over a 6-week period in both groups. Collagen was significantly increased and melanin significantly reduced in the silicone gel group compared with the placebo group. Positive results in both groups is possible. Larger controlled studies are required in order to evaluate this treatment further.

Trofolastin cream is a topical preparation that is used as prophylactic treatment and contains the active ingredients *Centella asiatica* tocopherol and collagen-elastin hydrolysates.[84] The mechanism of action is to stimulate fibroblasts and reduce the production of glucocorticoids.[84] It has been advocated that a small amount of cream to cover the area should be massaged daily into the skin.[90] In a double-blind trial (LOE-2) conducted by Mallol and colleagues,[90] Trofolastin and a placebo cream were applied to 80 pregnant women of varying ethnicities with SD for 6 months. Eighty-nine percent of women in the treated group did not develop SD compared with 100% in the placebo group. However, there was no description regarding group allocation. In addition, 20% of the participants withdrew from the study, which could have affected these results.

Light Therapy

Light therapy has been used for treating SD, HTS, and KD.[91–93] Photodynamic therapy (PDT) is a technique that uses light to activate a photosensitiser localized in diseased tissues.[93] PDT has been shown to reduce type I collagen synthesis and fibroblast proliferation in vitro.[91,92] The use of PDT was initially described in a case report (LOE-5) of a patient with a persistent keloid, and it showed positive effects.[92] Following 5 methyl aminolevulinate-PDT sessions, scar color had improved and the keloid had reduced in size and become flatter, with reduced erythema in the surrounding margin. Side effects of PDT include short-term pain and inflammation, as well as longer term hypopigmentation or hyperpigmentation.[92] Our team recently showed, in 20 patients of skin types II to VI, that 3 treatments of PDT (37 J/cm^2) at weekly intervals were effective in reducing pruritus, pain, and keloid volume, and increasing pliability of symptomatic keloid scars (LOE-3).[93] PDT is a promising treatment of KD in patients with dark pigmented skin. Nevertheless, more controlled studies are required to further evaluate the optimal PDT treatment regimen.

Intense pulsed light (IPL) is a noncoherent filtered flash-lamp emitting visible light with wavelengths of 515 to 1200 nm.[94] In a study by Hernández-Pérez and colleagues,[94] the use of IPL on striae albae was evaluated and there was a reduction in the number and length of SD.[94] Postinflammatory hyperpigmentation was noted in 40% of patients treated with IPL. Ultraviolet A (UVA)/ultraviolet B (UVB) therapy has also been used in the treatment of SD and has been shown to improve hypopigmentation.[95] In a prospective clinical study (LOE-4) evaluating the efficacy and safety of UVB/UVA1 therapy for striae albae, 14 participants with skin types II to VI were treated up to 10 times with the therapy.[95] This therapy was effective for short-term repigmentation of hypopigmented SD. However, only 9 participants completed all treatment visits so this may have affected the results. The most common side effect was erythema, which resolved when treatment ceased.[96]

Electrical Stimulation

Studies have shown that electrical stimulation (ES) can enhance tissue healing and, more recently, have shown its use in the treatment of abnormal raised dermal scarring.[97–99] Various forms of ES have been used to treat different conditions: direct and alternating currents are useful in treating diabetic foot ulcers, skin ulcers, and chronic wounds.[97] More recently, a device named the Fenzian system, which produces degenerate waves, has been used in the treatment of KD and HTS.[97,98] It has been used to alleviate the symptoms of pain, pruritus, and inflammation in 2 case series (LOE-4) conducted by our team.[97,98] In these studies, a range of patients with varying skin types (I–VI) were included and this modality effectively controlled their symptoms. Furthermore, a study investigating the effect of PDT on keloid fibroblasts with and without ES showed that ES enhanced the cytotoxic effects of PDT and could be used as a combined therapy.[99] It is postulated that this treatment can be beneficial in the treatment of KD and HTS because it may negate the need for long-term pain medications. Further studies with long-term follow-up plus histologic evidence before-and-after therapy may provide further information as to the usefulness of this treatment in the management of symptomatic abnormal skin scars.

Lasers

Various lasers have been evaluated for the improvement of HTS and keloids.[100] The proposed benefit is produced by selective photothermolysis in which direct energy is absorbed by oxyhemoglobin, which leads to thermal injury and reduced collagen.[101]

Multiple treatments are required in order to provide a good outcome.[68] Treatment sessions usually occur at intervals of 4 to 8 weeks with between 1 and 24 treatments advocated depending on the type of scar.[102,103] The wavelength, fluences, spot size, beam profile, and protocol all contribute to the long-term outcome of abnormal scarring.[104] Lasers are safe in individuals with dark pigmented skins, but hypopigmentation and hyperpigmentation can occur, and are permanent in some cases.[105] Side effects noted with laser therapy are itching and purpuric spots, which tend to resolve within 1 week.[105]

Positive results have been shown with the 585-nm pulsed dye laser (PDL), which uses a concentrated beam of light that targets blood vessels in the skin, for the treatment of immature HTS and keloids.[102,103] It has been suggested that PDL induces capillary destruction and alters local collagen production.[103] A prospective study (LOE-4) by Hernández-Pérez and colleagues[94] showed that PDL was also able to clinically and microscopically improve SD after treatment.[94] The PDL has shown significant improvements in appearance of SD and increases elastin content.[106] However, problems have arisen when using this on striae albae because hyperpigmentation has occurred.[107] Two to 6 treatment sessions have been suggested to improve scar height, color, pliability, and texture.[1] However, the results in some case-control studies (LOE-4) do not support this because of the lack of untreated control groups, length of follow-up being too short to note long-term differences, small sample sizes, and studies that combine HTS and KD.[67,102,103] Hyperpigmentation can occur, predominantly in darker skin types, but is less common with the use of the wavelength 595 nm than with 585 nm.[106]

Furthermore, the 1064-nm neodymium (Nd):yttrium aluminum garnet (YAG) laser has been used to improve KD and HTS.[108] It has been suggested that the Nd:YAG can reach deeper than the PDL and is able to treat larger, more dense KD.[108] However, its efficacy reduces with the thickness of the scar.[108,109] The Nd-YAG has also been used to treat patients with SD.[109] Goldman and colleagues[109] treated 20 patients with striae rubrae and showed positive outcomes, although these were based on subjective opinions of the doctors and the patients (LOE-5).[109]

The short-pulsed CO_2 laser has shown variable results in the treatment of SD.[110,111] Nouri and colleagues[110] showed that 4 patients with a Fitzpatrick skin type IV to VI developed postinflammatory hyperpigmentation.[110] However, Lee and colleagues[111] showed an improvement in SD in 27 patients of Asian descent with striae albae with skin type IV.[111]

Many of the studies that evaluate the efficacy of laser therapies in abnormal raised scarring and SD are of low quality because of problems with blinding and a lack of controls. It is important to be aware of the various types of lasers and their uses in treating SD, KD, and HTS in dark pigmented skin types to ensure safety and to identify significant side effects.

COMBINATION THERAPIES

There are various combination therapies that have been used to treat KD and HTS, although none of note for SD. Intralesional steroid injections have been combined with adjuvant therapies, such as surgical excision to beneficial effect.[112,113] A clinical review (LOE-4) showed that 18 patients with dark pigmented skin treated with core excision and delayed intralesional steroid injection were successfully treated without recurrence.[112] All patients were followed up for 2 years and the common side effect observed was hypopigmentation. Supporting this delayed intralesional steroid technique, Froelich and colleagues[114] suggest that early administration of steroids and excision can lead to wound dehiscence.

An RCT (LOE-1) examined the potential benefit of combining intralesional steroid with 5-FU in patients with KD in a double-blind trial.[38] Over a 3-month period, 40 patients of varying skin types received weekly injections of triamcinolone acetonide (40 mg/mL) or triamcinolone acetonide and 5-FU (50 mg/mL) for a total of 8 treatments. After 12 weeks, significant parameter improvements were observed in the steroid and 5-FU treatment arm compared with the steroid-alone arm.

SELF-MANAGEMENT STRATEGIES

Among obese individuals with a body mass index of 27 to 51, the prevalence of SD is reported to be 43%.[115] Individuals can take an active approach by maintaining a healthy diet to reduce excess weight gain. In addition, a randomized trial using topical treatment on SD noted that the positive effects observed may have occurred secondary to topical massage because no placebo group was included.[116]

There is limited evidence that shows how massage affects the skin,[117,118] although anecdotally it is recommended that patients presenting with scars should massage to improve the quality.[119,120] There are suggestions that the efficacy of massage is greater in postsurgical scars.[118] A review on the role of massage in scar management by Shin and Bordeaux[118] suggested that the evidence available is weak, regimens are varied, and the outcomes are difficult to standardize.

SURGICAL TREATMENT OPTIONS AND PROCEDURE

Surgery is a common management strategy for KD and HTS (**Box 1**). However, there are no widely accepted surgical procedures used in the treatment of SD. In relation to HTS, surgical intervention is common, especially in the case of HTS caused by burns when contractures need to be released.[5] KD has 2 main objectives: to resect or debulk. Because keloid excision at high risk of recurrence, it is important to construct a management plan that includes adjuvant therapy following surgery.[29] There are various types of surgical excisions used to improve and revise KD and HTS, such as Z-plasty; W-plasty; linear closure; excision with grafting; and, as a final option, flap coverage.[40] The operating surgeon should be aware that the margin of the KD has been found to be highly active,[75] and, when excising a scar, Tan and colleagues[121] showed the benefit of extralesional removal of the scar to reduce the risk of recurrence. Serial scar excision has been advocated for larger KD, for which intralesional procedures are used on numerous occasions to reduce skin tension before using an extralesional technique.[122,123] Surgical incisions along the line of tension and closure without tension are of paramount importance.[124] Furthermore, core excision of KD in which the epidermis and partial dermal layer resurface the defect has also been used by others.[125]

Intralesional excisions of HTS facial scars have also provided good aesthetic results,[125] and KD flap core excision procedures have shown no

recurrence after the absence of adjuvant therapy in 2 case-series studies (LOE-4).[126] A randomised, prospective study (LOE-2) investigated the usefulness of surgical excision alone, surgical excision and intralesional steroid, and surgical excision and radiotherapy in 42 patients with 50 earlobe KD.[127] The results showed no statistically significant differences between each group; however, these results may have been affected by the dropout of 11 patients.

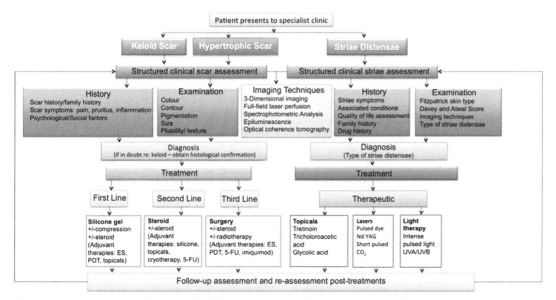

Fig. 5. The management pathway for keloid scars, hypertrophic scars and striae distensae.

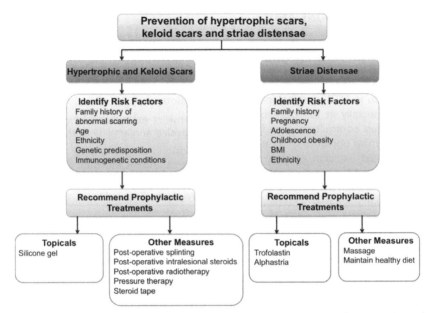

Fig. 6. The prevention of hypertrophic scars, keloid scars, and SD including the risk factors and prophylactic treatments available.

The most appropriate incision design must be selected, according to the shape of scar, its anatomic location, and the degree of contracture. V-Y flaps may be suited to the correction of cutaneous facial defects, and although W-plasty is effective in most linear scars, it is less useful for wide or raised scars.[69] Suture materials have been advocated in areas of high tension such as the sternum. RCTs comparing absorbable with suture materials have not found any significant differences in the long-term cosmetic outcomes.[128,129]

TREATMENT RESISTANCE

The management of KD and HTS, in particular, is especially difficult because of the considerably high rate of recurrence. Studies frequently assess the outcome parameter of scar recurrence but no clear definition of this subjective parameter is defined.[40] Bayat and colleagues[130] studied the clinical characteristics of 211 Afro-Caribbean patients with KD and noted that young female patients ($P<.001$) and those with a positive family history ($P<.002$) of KD were associated with the development of KD in multiple anatomic sites. Therefore, this is of importance in predicting KD response to treatment and prognosis and in identifying those at higher risk of disease recurrence.

EVALUATION OF OUTCOME AND LONG-TERM RECOMMENDATIONS

It is essential to ensure that a strategic approach is made to fully assess a patient in order to create

a patient-specific management/treatment plan (**Fig. 5**). A focused history regarding the patient, physically, psychologically, and socially, should provide a direct approach for targeted therapy with reevaluation and follow-up occurring on a regular basis. Targeting the patient's main symptoms and needs ensures that their concerns are met and are used as the focus for treatment strategies. In addition, prevention should be the main focus in order to prophylactically treat the KD, HTS, or SD (**Fig. 6**).

SUMMARY

Problematic abnormal scars and SD in dark pigmented skin are difficult to eradicate and most of the modalities available are associated with some adverse side effects. The evidence for recommended treatment options are at best variable and often limited, because most published studies have limited follow-up, subjective evaluation of treatment outcome, and poor study design. Many studies do not differentiate between KD and HTS, because HTS tends to respond better to more simple treatments. New emerging therapies such as PDT and ES have shown promise in the treatment of HTS and KD and in patients with dark pigmented skin, although further studies are needed to elucidate the effectiveness. There are many treatment options for SD, prophylactic and therapeutic, but they have shown variable results. Moreover, the prevention of KD, HTS, and SD is paramount and, in particular for KD, combination therapy tends to be the most effective rather than single treatment modalities. Further high-quality research is needed to identify effective treatments for patients with dark pigmented skin and to tailor these treatments to each individual.

REFERENCES

1. Alster TS, Handrick C. Laser treatment of hypertrophic scars, keloids, and striae. Semin Cutan Med Surg 2000;19:287–92.
2. Gauglitz GG. Management of keloids and hypertrophic scars: current and emerging options. Clin Cosmet Investig Dermatol 2013;6:103–14.
3. Thomas RG, Liston WA. Clinical associations of striae gravidarum. J Obstet Gynaecol 2004;24: 270–1.
4. Murray JC. Keloids and hypertrophic scars. Clin Dermatol 1994;12:27.
5. Bayat A, McGrouther DA, Ferguson MW. Skin scarring. BMJ 2003;326:88–92.
6. Ud-Din S, Bayat A. Strategic management of keloid disease in ethnic skin: a structured approach supported by the emerging literature. Br J Dermatol 2013;169(Suppl 3):71–81.
7. Bloemen MC, van der Veer WM, Ulrich MM, et al. Prevention and curative management of hypertrophic scar formation. Burns 2009;35:463–75.
8. Al-Attar A, Mess S, Thomassen JM, et al. Keloid pathogenesis and treatment. Plast Reconstr Surg 2006;117:286–300.
9. Datubo-Brown D. Keloids: a review of the literature. Br J Plast Surg 1990;43:70–7.
10. Bock O, Schmid-Ott G, Malewski P, et al. Quality of life of patients with keloid and hypertrophic scarring. Arch Dermatol Res 2006;297:433–8.
11. Brown JJ, Bayat A. Genetic susceptibility to raised dermal scarring. Br J Dermatol 2006;161:8–18.
12. Kang S. Topical tretinoin therapy for management of early striae. J Am Acad Dermatol 1998;39:90–2.
13. Kharb S, Gundgurthi A, Dutta MK, et al. Striae atrophicans: a mimic to Cushing's cutaneous striae. Indian J Endocrinol Metab 2012;16(Suppl 1):S123.
14. Rogalski C, Haustein UF, Glander HJ, et al. Extensive striae distensae as a result of topical corticosteroid therapy in psoriasis vulgaris. Acta Derm Venereol 2003;83:54–5.
15. Elson ML. Topical tretinoin in the treatment of striae distensae and in the promotion of wound healing: a review. J Dermatolog Treat 1994;5:163–5.
16. Hermanns JF, Piérard GE. High-resolution epiluminescence colorimetry of striae distensae. J Eur Acad Dermatol Venereol 2006;20:282–7.
17. Cho S, Park ES, Lee DH, et al. Clinical features and risk factors for striae distensae in Korean adolescents. J Eur Acad Dermatol Venereol 2006;20: 1108–13.
18. Elbuluk N, Kang S, Hamilton T. Differences in clinical features and risk factors for striae distensae in African American and white women. J Am Acad Dermatol 2009;60(Suppl 1):AB56.
19. Moncrieff M, Cotton S, Claridge E, et al. Spectrophotometric intracutaneous analysis: a new technique for imaging pigmented skin lesions. Br J Dermatol 2002;146:448–57.
20. Pierard-Franchimont C, Hermanns JF, Hermanns-Le T, et al. Striae distensae in darker skin types: the influence of melanocyte mechanobiology. J Cosmet Dermatol 2005;4:174–8.
21. Dusch M, Schley M, Rukwied R, et al. Rapid flare development evoked by current frequency-dependent stimulation analyzed by full-field laser perfusion imaging. Neuroreport 2007;18:1101–5.
22. Perry D, McGrouther DA, Bayat A. Current tools for non-invasive objective assessment of skin scars. Plast Reconstr Surg 2010;126:912–23.
23. Bleve M, Capra P, Pavanetto F, et al. Ultrasound and 3D skin imaging: methods to evaluate efficacy of striae distensae treatment. Dermatol Res Pract 2012;2012:1–10.
24. Hambleton J, Shakespeare PG, Pratt BJ. The progress of hypertrophic scars monitored by ultrasound measurements of thickness. Burns 1992; 18:301–7.
25. Corica GF, Wigger NC, Edgar DW, et al. Objective measurement of scarring by multiple assessors: is the tissue tonometer a reliable option? J Burn Care Res 2006;27:520–3.
26. Gupta V, Gupta A, Gogra MR. Optical coherence tomography of macular diseases. New York: Taylor & Francis; 2004.
27. Oliveira GV, Hawkins HK, Chinkes D, et al. Hypertrophic versus non-hypertrophic scars compared by immunohistochemistry and laser confocal microscopy: type I and III collagens. Int Wound J 2009;6:445–52.
28. Rolfe H, Wurm E, Gilmore S. An investigation of striae distensae using reflectance confocal microscopy. Australas J Dermatol 2012;53:181–5.
29. Mustoe TA, Cooter RD, Gold MH. International clinical recommendations on scar management. Plast Reconstr Surg 2002;110:560–71.
30. Mustoe TA. Evolution of silicone therapy and mechanism of action in scar management. Aesthetic Plast Surg 2008;32:82–92.
31. Griffith BH, Monroe CW, McKinney P. A follow-up study on the treatment of keloids with triamcinolone acetonide. Plast Reconstr Surg 1970;46:145–50.
32. Jalali M, Bayat A. Current use of steroids in management of abnormal raised skin scars. Surgeon 2007;5:175–80.
33. Cohen IK, Diegelmann RF, Johnson ML. Effect of corticosteroids on collagen synthesis. Surgery 1977;82:15–20.

34. Kauh YC, Rouda S, Mondragon G, et al. Major suppression of pro-alpha1(I) type I collagen gene expression in the dermis after keloid excision and immediate intrawound injection of triamcinolone acetonide. J Am Acad Dermatol 1997;37:586–9.

35. Gauglitz GG, Korting HC, Pavicic T, et al. Hypertrophic scarring and keloids: pathomechanisms and current and emerging treatment strategies. J Mol Med 2011;17:113–25.

36. Berman B, Patel JK, Perez OA, et al. Evaluating the tolerability and efficacy of etanercept compared to triamcinolone acetonide for the intralesional treatment of keloids. J Drugs Dermatol 2008;7:757–61.

37. Manuskiatti W, Fitzpatrick RE. Treatment response of keloidal and hypertrophic sternotomy scars: comparison among intralesional corticosteroid, 5-fluorouracil, and 585-nm flashlamp-pumped pulsed-dye laser treatments. Arch Dermatol 2002; 138:1149–55.

38. Darougheh A, Asilian A, Shariati F. Intralesional triamcinolone alone or in combination with 5-fluorouracil for the treatment of keloid and hypertrophic scars. Clin Exp Dermatol 2009;34:219–23.

39. Darzi MA, Chowdri NA, Kaul SK, et al. Evaluation of various methods of treating keloids and hypertrophic scars: a 10-year follow-up study. Br J Plast Surg 1992;45:374–9.

40. Reish RG, Eriksson E. Scars: a review of emerging and currently available therapies. Plast Reconstr Surg 2008;122:1068–78.

41. Ud-Din S, Bowring A, Derbyshire B, et al. Identification of steroid sensitive responders versus non-responders in the treatment of keloid disease. Arch Dermatol Res 2013;305:423–32.

42. Apikian M, Goodman G. Intralesional 5-fluorouracil in the treatment of keloid scars. Australas J Dermatol 2004;45:140–3.

43. Van Buskirk EM. Five-year follow-up of the Fluorouracil Filtering Surgery Study. Am J Ophthalmol 1996;122:751–2.

44. Fitzpatrick RE. Treatment of inflamed hypertrophic scars using intralesional 5-FU. Dermatol Surg 1999;25:224–32.

45. Kontochristopoulos G, Stefanaki C, Panagiotopoulos A, et al. Intralesional 5-fluorouracil in the treatment of keloids: an open clinical and histopathologic study. J Am Acad Dermatol 2005;52:474–9.

46. Khare N, Patil SB. A novel approach for management of ear keloids: results of excision combined with 5-fluorouracil injection. J Plast Reconstr Aesthet Surg 2012;65:315–7.

47. Hatamipour E, Mehrabi S, Hatamipour M, et al. Effects of combined intralesional 5-fluorouracil and topical silicone in prevention of keloids: a double blind randomized clinical trial study. Acta Med Iran 2011;49:127–30.

48. Sadeghinia A, Sadheginia S. Comparison of the efficacy of intralesional triamcinolone acetonide and 5-fluorouracil tattooing for the treatment of keloids. Dermatol Surg 2012;38:104–9.

49. Nanda S, Reddy BS. Intralesional 5-fluorouracil as a treatment modality of keloids. Dermatol Surg 2004;30:54–6 [discussion: 56–7].

50. Gupta S, Kalra A. Efficacy and safety of intralesional 5-fluorouracil in the treatment of keloids. Dermatology 2002;204:130–2.

51. Goldan O, Weissman O, Regev E, et al. Treatment of postdermabrasion facial hypertrophic and keloid scars with intralesional 5-fluorouracil injections. Aesthetic Plast Surg 2008;32:389–92.

52. Kang S, Kim KJ, Griffiths CE, et al. Topical tretinoin (retinoic acid) improves early stretch marks. Arch Dermatol 1996;132:519–26.

53. Rangel O, Arias I, Garcia E, et al. Topical tretinoin 0.1% for pregnancy related abdominal striae: an open-label, multicenter, prospective study. Adv Ther 2001;18:181–6.

54. Pribanich S, Simpson FG, Held B, et al. Low-dose tretinoin does not improve striae distensae: a double-blind, placebo-controlled study. Cutis 1994; 54:121–4.

55. Elson ML. Treatment of striae distensae with topical tretinoin. J Dermatol Surg Oncol 1990;16:267–70.

56. Ash K, Lord J, Zukowski M, et al. Comparison of topical therapy for striae alba (20% glycolic acid/ 0.05% tretinoin versus 20% glycolic acid/10% L-ascorbic acid). Dermatol Surg 1998;24:849–56.

57. Kim SJ, Park JH, Kim DH, et al. Increased in vivo collagen synthesis and in vitro cell proliferative effect of glycolic acid. Dermatol Surg 1998;24:1054–8.

58. Adatto MA, Deprez P. Striae treated by a novel combination treatment–sand abrasion and a patent mixture containing 15% trichloracetic acid followed by 6-24 hrs of a patent cream under plastic occlusion. J Cosmet Dermatol 2003;2:61–7.

59. Obagi ZE, Obagi S, Alaiti S, et al. TCA-based blue peel: a standardized procedure with depth control. Dermatol Surg 1999;25:773–80.

60. Mazzarello V, Farace F, Ena P, et al. A superficial texture analysis of 70% glycolic acid topical therapy and striae distensae. Plast Reconstr Surg 2012;129:589–90.

61. Perkins K, Davey RB, Wallis KA. Silicone gel: a new treatment for burn scars and contractures. Burns 1983;9:201–4.

62. Chan KY, Lau CL, Adeeb SM, et al. A randomized, placebo-controlled, double-blind, prospective clinical trial of silicone gel in prevention of hypertrophic scar development in median sternotomy wound. Plast Reconstr Surg 2005;116:1013–20 [discussion: 1012–21].

63. Berman B, Flores F. Comparison of a silicone gel-filled cushion and silicon gel sheeting for the

63. treatment of hypertrophic or keloid scars. Dermatol Surg 1999;25:484–6.

64. Sawada Y, Sone K. Treatment of scars and keloids with a cream containing silicone oil. Br J Plast Surg 1990;43:683–8.

65. Stoffels I, Wolter TP, Sailer AM, et al. The impact of silicone spray on scar formation. A single-center placebo-controlled double-blind trial. Hautarzt 2010;61:332–8.

66. Palmieri B, Gozzi G, Palmieri G. Vitamin E added silicone gel sheets for treatment of hypertrophic scars and keloids. Int J Dermatol 1995;34:506–9.

67. Durani P, Bayat A. Levels of evidence for the treatment of keloid disease. J Plast Reconstr Aesthet Surg 2008;61:4–17.

68. Sawada Y, Sone K. Hydration and occlusion treatment for hypertrophic scars and keloids. Br J Plast Surg 1992;45:599–603.

69. Chang CC, Kuo YF, Chiu HC, et al. Hydration, not silicone, modulates the effects of keratinocytes on fibroblasts. J Surg Res 1995;59:705–11.

70. Majan JI. Evaluation of a self-adherent soft silicone dressing for the treatment of hypertrophic postoperative scars. J Wound Care 2006;15:193–6.

71. Lee SM, Ngim CK, Chan YY, et al. A comparison of Sil-K and Epiderm in scar management. Burns 1996;22:483–7.

72. Nikkonen MM, Pitkanen JM, Al-Qattan MM. Problems associated with the use of silicone gel sheeting for hypertrophic scars in the hot climate of Saudi Arabia. Burns 2001;27:498–501.

73. Rayatt S, Subramaniyan V, Smith G. Audit of reactions to topical silicon used in the management of hypertrophic scars. Burns 2006;32:653–4.

74. de Oliveira GV, Nunes TA, Magna LA, et al. Silicone versus nonsilicone gel dressings: a controlled trial. Dermatol Surg 2001;27:721–6.

75. Ogawa R. The most current algorithms for the treatment and prevention of hypertrophic scars and keloids. Plast Reconstr Surg 2010;125:557–68.

76. O'Brien L, Pandit A. Silicon gel sheeting for preventing and treating hypertrophic and keloid scars. Cochrane Database Syst Rev 2006;(1):CD003826.

77. Yosipovitch G, Widijanti Sugeng M, Goon A, et al. A comparison of the combined effect of cryotherapy and corticosteroid injections versus corticosteroids and cryotherapy alone on keloids: a controlled study. J Dermatolog Treat 2001;12:87–90.

78. Rusciani L, Rossi G, Bono R. Use of cryotherapy in the treatment of keloids. J Dermatol Surg Oncol 1993;19:529–34.

79. Zouboulis CC, Zouridaki E, Rosenberger A, et al. Current developments and uses of cryosurgery in the treatment of keloids and hypertrophic scars. Wound Repair Regen 2002;10:98–102.

80. Lahiri A, Tsiliboti D, Gaze NR. Experience with difficult keloids. Br J Plast Surg 2001;54:633–5.

81. Layton AM, Yip J, Cunliffe WJ. A comparison of intralesional triamcinolone and cryosurgery in the treatment of acne keloids. Br J Dermatol 1994; 130:498–501.

82. Fikrle T, Pizinger K. Cryosurgery in the treatment of earlobe keloids: report of seven cases. Dermatol Surg 2005;31:1728–31.

83. Gupta S, Kumar B. Intralesional cryosurgery using lumbar puncture and/or hypodermic needles for large, bulky, recalcitrant keloids. Int J Dermatol 2001;40:349–53.

84. Brinkhaus B, Lindner M, Schuppan D, et al. Chemical, pharmacological and clinical profile of the East Asian medical plant *Centella asiatica*. Phytomedicine 2000;7:427–48.

85. Shah DN, Recktenwall-Work SM, Anseth KS. The effect of bioactive hydrogels on the secretion of extracellular matrix molecules by valvular interstitial cells. Biomaterials 2008;29:2060–72.

86. de Buman M, Walther M, de Weck R. Effectiveness of Alphastria cream in the prevention of pregnancy stretch marks (striae distensae). Results of a double-blind study. Gynakol Rundsch 1987;27: 79–84.

87. Young G, Jewell D. Creams for preventing stretch marks in pregnancy. Cochrane Database Syst Rev 1996;(2):CD000066.

88. Brennan M, Young G, Devane D, et al. Topical preparations for preventing stretch marks in pregnancy. Cochrane Database Syst Rev 2012;(11):CD000066.

89. Ud-Din S, McAnelly SL, Bowring A, et al. A double-blind controlled clinical trial assessing the effect of topical gels on striae distensae (stretch marks): a non-invasive imaging, morphological and immunohistochemical study. Arch Dermatol Res 2013; 305(7):1–15.

90. Mallol J, Belda MA, Costa D, et al. Prophylaxis of striae gravidarum with a topical formulation. A double blind trial. Int J Cosmet Sci 1991;13:51–7.

91. Mendoza J, Sebastian A, Allan E, et al. Differential cytotoxic response in keloid fibroblasts exposed to photodynamic therapy is dependent on photosensitiser precursor, fluence and location of fibroblasts within the lesion. Arch Dermatol Res 2012;304: 549–62.

92. Nie Z, Bayat A, Behzad F, et al. Positive response of a recurrent keloid scar to topical methyl aminolevulinate-photodynamic therapy. Photodermatol Photoimmunol Photomed 2010;26:330–2.

93. Ud-Din S, Thomas G, Morris J, et al. Photodynamic therapy: an innovative approach to the treatment of keloid disease evaluated using subjective and objective non-invasive tools. Arch Dermatol Res 2013;305:205–14.

94. Hernández-Pérez E, Colombo-Charrier E, Valencia-Ibiett E. Intense pulsed light in the treatment

of striae distensae. Dermatol Surg 2002;28:1124–30.

95. Sadick NS, Magro C, Hoenig A. Prospective clinical and histological study to evaluate the efficacy and safety of a targeted high-intensity narrow band UVB/UVA1 therapy for striae alba. J Cosmet Laser Ther 2007;9:79–83.

96. Goldberg DJ, Marmur ES, Schmults C, et al. Histologic and ultrastructural analysis of ultraviolet B laser and light source treatment of leukoderma in striae distensae. Dermatol Surg 2005; 31:385–7.

97. Ud-Din S, Giddings P, Colthurst J, et al. Significant reduction of symptoms of scarring with electrical stimulation: evaluated with subjective and objective assessment tools. Wounds 2013;25:212–24.

98. Perry D, Colthurst J, Giddings P, et al. Treatment of symptomatic abnormal skin scars with electrical stimulation. J Wound Care 2010;19:447–53.

99. Sebastian A, Allan E, Allan D, et al. Addition of novel degenerate electrical waveform stimulation with photodynamic therapy significantly enhances its cytotoxic effect in keloid fibroblasts: first report of a potential combination therapy. J Dermatol Sci 2011;64:174–84.

100. Apfelberg DB, Maser MR, Lash H, et al. Preliminary results of argon and carbon dioxide laser treatment of keloid scars. Lasers Surg Med 1984; 4:283–90.

101. Reiken SR, Wolfort SF, Berthiaume F, et al. Control of hypertrophic scar growth using selective photothermolysis. Lasers Surg Med 1997;21:7–12.

102. Paquet P, Hermanns JF, Pierard GE. Effect of the 585nm flashlamp-pumped pulsed dye laser for the treatment of keloids. Dermatol Surg 2001;27:171–4.

103. Wittenberg GP, Fabian BG, Bogomillsky JL, et al. Prospective, singleblind, randomized, controlled study to assess the efficacy of the 585nm flashlamp-pumped pulsed dye laser and silicone gel sheeting in hypertrophic scar treatment. Arch Dermatol 1999;135:1049–55.

104. Jackson BA, Arndt KA, Dover JS. Are all 585nm pulsed dye lasers equivalent: a prospective, comparative, photometric histological study. J Am Acad Dermatol 1996;34:1000–4.

105. Manuskiatti W, Wanitphakdeedecha R, Fitzpatrick RE. Effect of pulse width of a 595-nm flashlamp-pumped pulsed dye laser on the treatment response of keloidal and hyper-trophic sternotomy scars. Dermatol Surg 2007;33:152–61.

106. McDaniel DH, Ash K, Zukowski M. Treatment of stretch marks with the 585-nm flashlamp-pumped pulsed dye laser. Dermatol Surg 1996;22:332–7.

107. Jimenez GP, Flores F, Berman B, et al. Treatment of striae rubra and striae alba with the 585-nm pulsed-dye laser. Dermatol Surg 2003;29:362–5.

108. Akaishi S, Koike S, Dohi T, et al. Nd:YAG laser treatment of keloids and hypertrophic scars. Eplasty 2012;12:e1.

109. Goldman A, Rossato F, Prati C. Stretch marks: treatment using the 1,064-nm Nd:YAG laser. Dermatol Surg 2008;34:686–92.

110. Nouri K, Romagosa R, Chartier T, et al. Comparison of the 585 nm pulse dye laser and the short pulsed CO_2 laser in the treatment of striae distensae in skin types IV and VI. Dermatol Surg 1999;25:368–70.

111. Lee SE, Kim JH, Lee SJ, et al. Treatment of striae distensae using an ablative 10,600nm carbon dioxide fractional laser: a retrospective review of 27 participants. Dermatol Surg 2010;36:1683–90.

112. Donkor P. Head and neck keloid: treatment by core excision and delayed intralesional injection of steroid. J Oral Maxillofac Surg 2007;65:1292–6.

113. Roques C, Teot L. The use of corticosteroids to treat keloids: a review. Int J Low Extrem Wounds 2008;7:137–45.

114. Froelich K, Staudenmaier R, Kleinsasser N, et al. Therapy of auricular keloids: review of different treatment modalities and proposal for a therapeutic algorithm. Eur Arch Otorhinolaryngol 2007;264:1497–508.

115. García-Hidalgo L, Orozco-Topete R, Gonzalez-Barranco J, et al. Dermatoses in 156 obese adults. Obes Res 1999;7:299–302.

116. Wierrani F, Kozak W, Schramm W, et al. Attempt of preventive treatment of striae gravidarum using preventive massage ointment administration. Wien Klin Wochenschr 1992;104:42–4.

117. Rapaport MH, Schettler P, Bresee C. A preliminary study of the effects of a single session of Swedish massage on the hypothalamic-pituitary-adrenal and immune function in normal individuals. J Altern Complement Med 2010;16:1–10.

118. Shin TM, Bordeaux JS. The role of scar management: a literature review. Dermatol Surg 2012;38:414–23.

119. Roques C. Massage applied to scars. Wound Repair Regen 2002;10:126–8.

120. Holavanahalli RK, Helm PA, Parry IS. Select practices in management and rehabilitation of burns: a survey report. J Burn Care Res 2011;32:210–23.

121. Tan K, Shah N, Pritchard S, et al. The influence of surgical excision margins on keloid prognosis. Ann Plast Surg 2010;64:55–8.

122. Stahl S, Barnea Y, Weiss J, et al. Treatment of earlobe keloids by extralesional excision combined with preoperative and post-operative "sandwich" radiotherapy. Plast Reconstr Surg 2010;125:135–41.

123. Akaishi S, Akimoto M, Ogawa R, et al. The relationship between keloid growth pattern and stretching tension: visual analysis using the finite element method. Ann Plast Surg 2008;60:445–51.

124. Meyer M, McGrouther DA. A study relating wound tension to scar morphology in the pre-sternal scar using Langers technique. Br J Plast Surg 1991; 44:291–4.

125. Ziccardi VB, Lamphier J. Use of keloid skin as an autograft for earlobe reconstruction after excision. Oral Surg Oral Med Oral Pathol Oral Radiol Endod 2000;89:674–5.

126. Lee Y, Minn KW, Baek RM, et al. A new surgical treatment of keloid: keloid core excision. Ann Plast Surg 2001;46:135–40.

127. Sclafani AP, Gordon L, Chadha M, et al. 3rd Prevention of earlobe keloid recurrence with postoperative corticosteroid injections versus radiation therapy: a randomized, prospective study and review of the literature. Dermatol Surg 1996; 22:569–74.

128. Parell GJ, Becker GD. Comparison of absorbable with nonabsorbable sutures in closure of facial skin wounds. Arch Facial Plast Surg 2003;5:488–90.

129. Sanders KW, Gage-White L, Stucker FJ. Topical mitomycin C in the prevention of keloid scar recurrence. Arch Facial Plast Surg 2005;7:172–5.

130. Bayat A, Arscott G, Ollier WE, et al. Keloid disease: clinical relevance of single versus multiple site scars. Br J Plast Surg 2005;58:28–37.

The Spectrum of HIV-Associated Infective and Inflammatory Dermatoses in Pigmented Skin

Mojakgomo Hendrick Motswaledi, MBChB, MMED(Derm), FCDerm(SA)[a],*,
Willie Visser, MBChB, MFamMed, MMED(Derm)[b]

KEYWORDS

- Aids • HIV • Immunosuppression • Infections • Inflammatory dermatoses • Treatment

KEY POINTS

- The introduction of antiretroviral medication has changed the epidemiology, morbidity, and mortality of HIV disease.
- Antiretrovirals have also altered the incidence of infective and inflammatory diseases affecting the skin.
- Cutaneous disorders due to HIV infection remain a major problem in HIV-infected patients.
- In patients with pigmented skin, HIV-associated dermatoses result in special challenges, particularly with regard to diagnosis and treatment.
- Due to the common problem of dyspigmentation caused by these conditions in pigmented skin, early diagnosis and effective treatment are of utmost importance.

INTRODUCTION

Patients living with HIV and AIDS are susceptible to various infective and inflammatory dermatoses. Even after the introduction of antiretroviral medication, the visible impact of skin lesions remains a major area of concern in patients living with HIV,[1] affecting their quality of life and self-esteem. In patients with pigmented skin, postinflammatory hyperpigmentation is a common finding and may lead to stigmatization and misdiagnosis.

Inflammatory and infective dermatoses can affect patients at any stage of HIV disease, with some considered markers of immunosuppression.

Skin lesions can predict treatment response or failure of antiretroviral medication; some worsen or appear initially after the initiation of antiretrovirals due to the immune reconstitution inflammatory syndrome (IRIS). Introduction of antiretroviral medication has changed the profile of HIV-associated dermatoses.[2] There is a dramatic decrease in opportunistic infections, whereas certain inflammatory conditions are on the increase.

In the setting of HIV/AIDS, it is important for physicians to be aware that infective and inflammatory dermatoses are often atypical, more severe, and more resistant to treatment.[1,3] There is a paucity of literature on HIV-associated skin disorders

Sponsorship: None.
Conflict of Interests: None.
[a] Department of Dermatology, University of Limpopo (Medunsa Campus), PO Box 1911, Medunsa, Pretoria 0204, South Africa; [b] Division of Dermatology, Department of Medicine, University of Stellenbosch, Cape Town, South Africa
* Corresponding author.
E-mail address: motswaledi1@webmail.co.za

in pigmented skin, especially in Africans. This article focuses on the clinical presentation in patients with pigmented skin of the most common HIV-associated infective and inflammatory dermatoses.

VIRAL INFECTIONS
Herpes Simplex Virus Infection

Herpes simplex virus (HSV) infection causes substantial morbidity in patients with HIV. HSV can serve as a cofactor in the progression of HIV.[4] This is suggested by simultaneous isolation of HSV and HIV from the same lesion, reduction of HIV shedding in coinfected individuals undertaking antiherpetic treatment, and data suggesting that HSV infection may adversely affect the progression of immunodeficiency in HIV-infected persons.[4] Herpes labialis caused by HSV type 1 (HSV-1) is common in HIV. In the setting of HIV, it tends to be more aggressive and lesions tend to last longer (**Fig. 1**). Herpes genitalis caused by HSV type 2 (HSV-2) is the most frequent genital ulcer disease among HIV seropositive patients.[4] Herpes genitalis presents as vesicles, erosions, and ulcers on the genitalia. In patients with AIDS, the severity and duration of recurrent genital herpes may be more severe than that seen in normal hosts.[4]

Molluscum Contagiosum

Molluscum contagiosum caused by a poxvirus is common in HIV. Lesions are skin-colored, dome-shaped papules or nodules with central umbilication.

In the setting of HIV, molluscum contagiosum tends to be atypical and extensive (**Fig. 2**). Atypical lesions may resemble other conditions, such as basal cell carcinoma, keratoacanthomas, and cryptococcosis. Although it is a clinical diagnosis, biopsy may be necessary to confirm the diagnosis. Histopathology shows intracytoplasmic inclusion

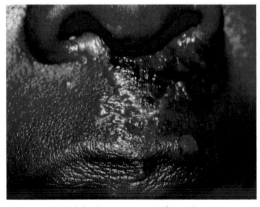

Fig. 1. Herpes labialis is an HIV-infected patient.

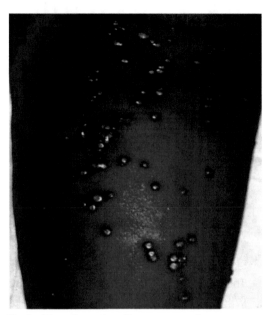

Fig. 2. Disseminated molluscum contagiosum.

bodies, called molluscum bodies or Henderson-Paterson bodies.

Treatment of molluscum contagiosum in HIV patients includes restoration of immune competence by highly active antiretroviral therapy.

In some patients, lesions may respond to immunomodulators, such as imiquimod 5% cream. Resistant lesions may be treated with cryotherapy, which involves application of liquid nitrogen onto the lesions for cold-induced cell destruction; however, this may not be possible in patients with extensive disease. Complications of cryotherapy are hypopigmentation, hyperpigmentation, and scarring.

Herpes Zoster

Herpes zoster is also common in HIV setting and tends to be multidermatomal (**Fig. 3**). HIV patients often get recurrent episodes. It presents as painful blisters after a dermatome. The pain may be severe in some patients and they are more likely to require medical attention.

Treatment of herpes zoster is aimed at speedy healing of skin lesions, limiting disease progression, pain reduction, and prevention of complications, such as postherpetic neuralgia.

Systemic antivirals, such as oral acyclovir (800 mg 5 times a day for 7–10 days) or valacyclovir (1000 mg 3 times a day for 7 days), are helpful. A combination of analgesics and antiinflammatories should be given for pain.

A common complication of herpes zoster is postherpetic neuralgia, in which the pain of herpes

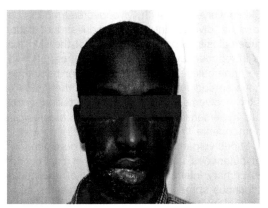

Fig. 3. Herpes zoster on maxillary and mandibular divisions of trigerminal nerve.

zoster remains long after the skin disease has healed. Management of postherpetic neuralgia includes analgesics, antiinflammatories, and a tricyclic antidepressant, such as amitriptyline. Antiepileptics, such as carbamazepine, can also be used instead of amitriptyline.

Viral Warts

Human papillomavirus warts are also common in HIV patients. They tend to be multiple in these patients. They can present in the form of verruca vulgaris or verruca plana. HIV patients with viral warts must be on antiretroviral therapy to boost the immune system.

Topical therapies, such as trichloroacetic acid and podophyllin resin in a compound tincture of benzoin, applied on to the lesions may help. Podophyllin acts by way of antimitotic activity. Immunomodulators, such as imiquimod 5% cream, may also be helpful.

Ablative therapies, such as cryotherapy and curettage, can also help in patients with fewer lesions. Long-pulsed Nd:YAG laser has also been used successfully in some patients.

BATERIAL INFECTIONS
Staphylococcus aureus Infection

Staphylococcus aureus is the most common bacterial pathogen in HIV. It causes folliculitis, impetigo, ecthyma, and skin abscesses. Treatment of staphylococcal skin disease includes the use of systemic antibiotics, such as cloxacillin, and application of topical antibiotics, such as mupirocin or fucidin. The use of antiseptic solutions in bath water may prevent recurrent episodes.

Bacillary Angiomatosis

Bacillary angiomatosis is a vascular proliferative disease common in HIV.[5] It is caused by Bartonella

henselae and Bartonella quintana. The proliferative vascular lesions most commonly involve the skin but may be present in many other tissues, including lymph nodes, bone, brain, respiratory and gastrointestinal tracts, cardiac valves, and bone marrow.[5]

It has been suggested that cutaneous lesions of bacillary angiomatosis may be a marker of systemic bacillary angiomatosis infection, especially in HIV-positive patients.[6] Cutaneous lesions of bacillary angiomatosis are angiomatous papules and nodules, which bleed easily on contact (**Fig. 4**). Treatment of choice is erythromycin (500 mg 4 times a day for 3 months). Doxycycline, ceftriaxone, and the fluoroquinolones can be useful.[6]

Syphilis

Syphilis is common in the setting of HIV, especially in HIV-positive men who have sex with men. Syphilis and HIV are particularly suited to being acquired together because both are sexually transmitted and the risk factors for acquisition are the same.[7,8] Furthermore, ulcers of primary syphilis are known to facilitate the transmission of HIV.[9,10]

In addition, syphilis has been reported to have immunologic effects on HIV infection, and HIV is known to modulate both the manifestations of syphilis and the serologic response to therapy.[7]

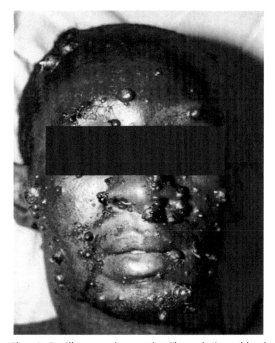

Fig. 4. Bacillary angiomatosis. These lesions bleed easily.

It has been postulated that the presentation of syphilis differs between HIV-infected patients and patients without HIV infection.

First, HIV-infected patients with primary syphilis are more likely to have multiple chancres compared with non-HIV patients.[8] In HIV patients, these ulcers tend to be larger and deeper.[10]

Second, HIV-infected patients with secondary syphilis frequently have simultaneous genital ulcers, thus have overlap of primary and secondary syphilis (**Fig. 5**).[8,10] It is unclear whether the overlapping of stages of syphilis in HIV patients represents slower than normal healing of primary syphilis or an accelerated progression to secondary syphilis.[8]

Third, HIV patients with syphilis have a higher likelihood of developing neurosyphilis.[8] In HIV patients with syphilis, atypical serologic tests and even serologically defined treatment failures have been reported.[11]

Cutaneous Tuberculosis

Cutaneous tuberculosis has re-emerged in areas with a high incidence of HIV infection and multidrug-resistant pulmonary tuberculosis.[12,13]

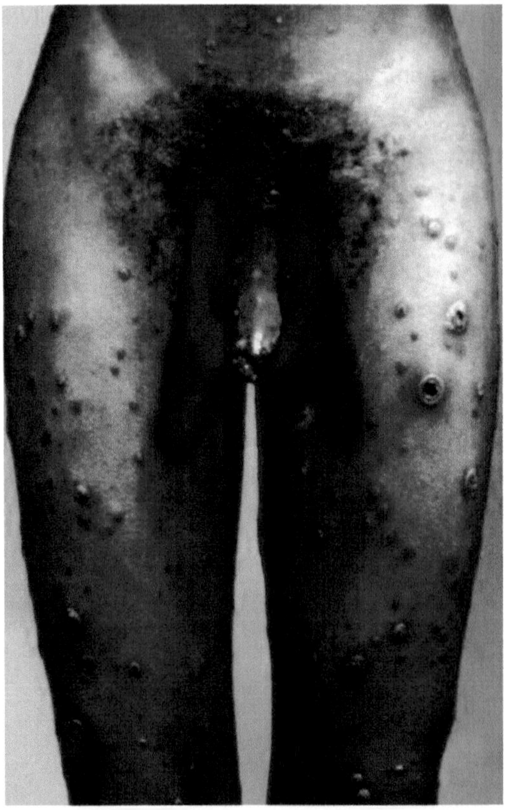

Skin involvement with *Mycobacterium tuberculosis* is divided into 3 categories: inoculation tuberculosis, a primary infection of the skin that is introduced by an exogenous source; secondary tuberculosis, either contiguous or hematogenous spread from a primary focus that leads to skin involvement; and, lastly, tuberculids, which are hypersensitivity reactions to *M tuberculosis* components.[14]

Lupus vulgaris remains the most common form of cutaneous tuberculosis,[12] and it can be due to primary infection of the skin or due to hematogenous spread. Lupus vulgaris presents as an asymptomatic enlarging plaque that later ulcerates and become verrucous, fungating, and destructive (**Fig. 6**). The nose and center of the face is a common area but any part of the body can be affected.

Scrofuloderma is another common form of cutaneous tuberculosis. It represents direct extension into the skin from an underlying tuberculosis focus, most commonly a lymph node or bone.

In HIV, dissemination of *M tuberculosis* to extrapulmonary sites, such as the skin, is more common, resulting in disseminated miliary tuberculosis of the skin, also known as tuberculosis cutis miliaris disseminata.[14] It is an uncommon form of tuberculosis characterized by a papulopustular eruption

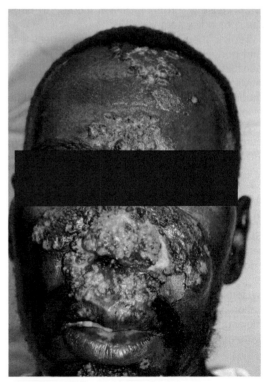

Fig. 5. Overlap of primary and secondary syphilis in an HIV patient.

Fig. 6. Verrucous, fungating lupus vulgaris on the face.

and hematogenous dissemination of tubercle bacilli to multiple organs, including the skin, and often has a poor prognosis.[15,16]

Papulonecrotic tuberculid occurs frequently in HIV patients. It is a symmetric eruption of necrotizing papules, appearing in crops and healing with scar formation (Fig. 7).[17] It is thought to be an immunologic response to *M tuberculosis* components in a previously sensitized patient after hematogenous spread from a focus of infection elsewhere.[18]

FUNGAL INFECTIONS
Dermatophytes

Both dermatophytes and deep fungal infections are common in HIV. They are a major source of morbidity and mortality. Dermatophytes infections are caused by fungi that invade the superficial dead layer of the skin as well as keratinized tissues, such as hair and nails. They occur commonly in temperate and tropical climates of Africa,[19,20] and HIV-positive patients are particularly susceptible. In a study by Petmy and colleagues[21] in Yaounde, Cameroon, 53% of HIV-positive patients were found to have at least 1 superficial fungal infection. The causative fungi are either geophilic, zoophilic, or anthropophilic, and they include *Epidermophyton floccosum, Microsporum canis, Trichophyton mentagrophytes, Trichophyton rubrum, Trichophyton tonsurans*, and *Trichophyton violaceum*.

Tinea corporis, tinea cruris, tinea pedis, and onychomycosis all occur commonly in patients with HIV infection.[22] Tinea cruris presents as an expanding scaling plaque of the upper thighs and groin with central clearing and an active border (Fig. 8). Tinea corporis in the setting of HIV disease virtually always is tinea cruris that has extended beyond the groin into the trunk.[22] In severely immunosuppressed patients with AIDS, lesions may have little inflammation and often lack the elevated border and central clearing typical of tinea.[22]

Onychomycosis is also common in HIV-positive patients. In non-HIV patients, the distal subungual pattern is the most common and occurs when the fungus invades the nail bed in the distal hyponychial area.

In HIV/AIDS patients, the proximal white subungual onychomycosis is the common type and is considered an early clinical marker of HIV infection.[22] In HIV patients, the clinical manifestations of dermatophyte infections may be atypical, making a diagnosis difficult. To ensure a correct diagnosis, skin scrapings should be collected for potassium hydroxide preparations and cultures.[22]

Dermatophyte infections in HIV respond well to topical antifungal agents. Systemic antifungals are reserved for extensive, chronic diseases.[22,23]

Deep Fungal Infections

Deep fungal infections, such as cryptococcosis and histoplasmosis, are also common in HIV patients.[24] *Cryptococcus neoformans* is a yeast with a predilection to the skin and the central nervous system. Cryptococcosis associated with HIV is common in Africa and Southeast Asia and is a frequent cause of death in patients with AIDS in these regions.[25]

Skin lesions occur in up to 10% of all patients with disseminated cryptococcosis and include

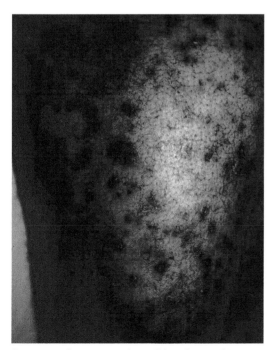

Fig. 7. Papulonecrotic tuberculid with atrophic scars.

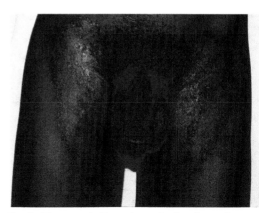

Fig. 8. Tinea cruris. Note the active border and central clearing.

papules, ulcerated nodules, subcutaneous nodules, Kaposi sarcoma–like lesions, and molluscum contangiosum–like lesions (**Fig. 9**).[25] Central nervous system involvement is common and occurs in 75% of HIV-infected patients with cryptococcosis. Unfortunately, symptoms and signs may be subtle, making early diagnosis difficult.[24] Ideally all patients with cutaneous cryptococcosis should have their cerebrospinal fluid examined because some patients may have cryptococcal meningitis with no symptoms and signs. Other areas that may be affected by cryptococcosis are the eyes, kidneys, prostate, adrenals, heart, liver, spleen, bone, muscles, and lymph nodes.[25]

Histoplasma capsulatum is a dimorphic fungus that grows as an intracellular yeast in the host and as a mold in vitro. It is also a common deep fungal infection. The etiologic agent of histoplasmosis associated with AIDS is *Histoplasma capsulatum* var. *capsulatum*.[25]

The clinical presentation includes fever, weight loss, hepatomegaly, splenomegaly, enteritis, chorioretinitis, endocarditis, meningitis, encephalitis, skin lesions, and pulmonary involvement.[24,25] Cutaneous involvement occurs in 11% of patients

owing to hematogenous dissemination from the pulmonary focus. Skin lesions are nonspecific and may be papules, patches, nodules, abscesses, plaques, pustules, and ulcers (**Fig. 10**).

Histology of the skin lesions may be diagnostic but the small size of organisms may elude easy detection. In disseminated disease, blood cultures and bone marrow cultures have the highest yield of organisms.

In treatment of both cryptococcosis and histoplasmosis, amphotericin B is the drug of choice. The initial induction therapy is generally amphotericin B, 0.5 to 1 mg/kg/d, followed by maintenance therapy with fluconazole or intraconazole.[24]

Treatment must be given for longer periods because recurrences are common in immunocompromised patients. Other deep fungal infections that can occur in HIV patients are coccidiomycosis, blastomycosis, paracoccidiomycosis, and sporotrichosis.[25]

PARASITIC INFESTATIONS

HIV patients often develop Norwegian scabies (crusted scabies), characterized by massive proliferation of *Sarcoptes scabiei* and highly

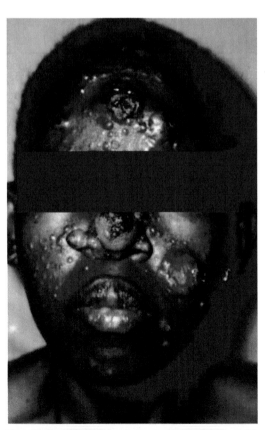

Fig. 9. Cryptococcosis in an HIV patient with meningitis.

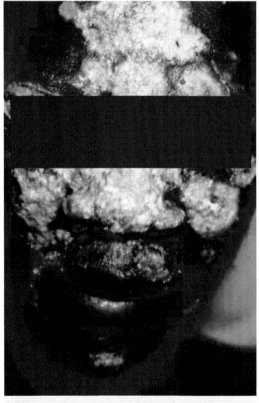

Fig. 10. Ulcerative lesions of histoplasmosis in an HIV patient.

contagious.[26] The combination of an atypical eruption and a high density of mites makes these patients a potential source of nosocomial scabies in hospitals and closed communities, such as residential homes.[26,27]

Clinically the lesions are generalized, hyperkeratotic scaly plaques that fall off easily (**Fig. 11**). Unlike in ordinary scabies, pruritus in Norwegian scabies is usually slight or absent.[26]

Although Norwegian scabies is a clinical diagnosis, there is often a delay in diagnosis because the cutaneous disease may resemble other scaly dermatoses that affect patients with AIDS, such as seborrheic dermatitis, psoriasis, or drug induced eruptions.[26] Early diagnosis is essential to prevent dissemination of this highly contagious form of scabies. Biopsy usually confirms the diagnosis. Unlike in ordinary scabies where mites or ova are difficult to find, in crusted scabies the stratum corneum is filled with these parasites (**Fig. 12**).

Patients' clothes and linens must be soaked and washed with hot water. Benzyl benzoate cream must be applied daily, but this is a skin irritant that may not be tolerated by children, in which case 10% sulfur in emulsifying ointment can be used. In many African countries where parasites

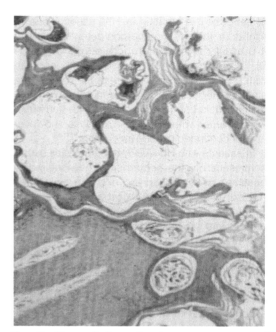

Fig. 12. Histopathology showing numerous ova of *Sarcoptes scabiei* (hematoxylin-eosin, original magnification ×40).

are a major problem, severe cases of Norwegian scabies are treated with intramuscular or oral ivermectin, but in South Africa, ivermectin is only registered for veterinary use.

INFLAMMATORY DERMATOSES
Seborrheic Dermatitis

Seborrheic dermatitis is a common chronic inflammatory dermatosis usually affecting infants before 3 to 6 months of age and adults at any age from puberty onwards.[28] This condition usually affects the sebaceous gland–rich areas of the body (ie, scalp, face, upper trunk, and skin folds).[29]

The incidence of seborrheic dermatitis in the general population is 2.35% to 11.3%.[30] In patients with HIV disease, the incidence increases to 30% to 80%, depending on the population studied.[31,32] In a recent study, seborrheic dermatitis was the second most frequent cutaneous finding in HIV-infected patients.[33]

The pathogenesis is the same as in immune-competent hosts and there is currently no consensus as to whether the growth of *Malassezia* yeasts on the skin of patients with HIV disease is increased or not.[34,35]

The subtype of *Malassezia* spp is thought to be different in HIV-positive individuals.[36] Immunologic factors play an important role in the pathogenesis of seborrheic dermatitis and may explain the increased incidence in HIV.[37] The clinical picture

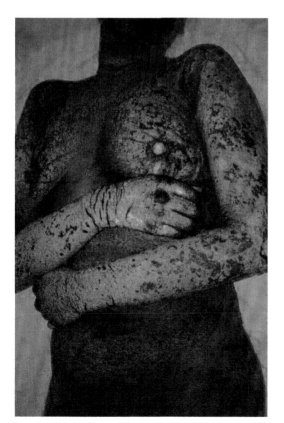

Fig. 11. Generalized Norwegian scabies in an HIV patient.

of seborrheic dermatitis in HIV patients can be similar to that in immune-competent hosts, but it is usually atypical and more severe (**Fig. 13**A, B).[31,38] The severity of the disease may correlate with the degree of immune suppression and the stage of HIV disease.[39,40] The increased severity of seborrheic dermatitis in HIV and the correlation with severity with advanced disease, however, are not confirmed by all investigators.[41,42]

In patients with HIV/AIDS, the dermatitis usually commences in the seborrheic areas but rapidly becomes more widespread and can even affect the extremities.[32] In Mali, seborrheic dermatitis was found a common presenting feature of HIV disease and can, therefore, be used as a predictor for HIV infection.[43]

The morphology can vary from that of acute dermatitis to psoriasiform plaques. In pigmented skin, seborrheic dermatitis can also present with annular hypopigmented patches, called petaloid seborrheic dermatitis. Erythema in pigmented skin is less visible and postlesional hyperpigmentation is common.

Due to the atypical presentation of seborrheic dermatitis in HIV disease, some investigators have argued that it should be considered to be a separate disease. The term, seborrheic-like dermatitis of AIDS, was proposed.[32] The histopathologic features and expression of heat shock proteins in seborrheic dermatitis in the setting of HIV are also different.[35,44] Any atypical presentation (more severe, atypical locations, and age distribution) of seborrheic dermatitis should alert clinicians to the possibility of HIV immunosuppression.

There are no clear guidelines for managing seborrheic dermatitis in the setting of HIV disease. The dermatitis is usually more resistant to treatment. The treatment consists of antifungal shampoos and creams, topical corticosteroids,[45] tacrolimus, or pimecrolimus in steroid-sensitive areas. Oral ketoconazole is often used in resistant cases.[46–48] Treating the underlying HIV/AIDS with antiretrovirals is important to control the disease, although this is not confirmed by all investigators.[1]

Psoriasis

The incidence of psoriasis in the general population is 2% to 3%. In HIV disease, the prevalence of psoriasis is usually the same or slightly increased.[49]

Psoriasis can be the presenting sign of HIV infection in some patients but can occur at any stage of HIV infection.[49] In the setting of HIV, psoriasis is usually more severe and the severity correlates with the degree of immunosuppression (**Fig. 14**).[50]

HIV disease frequently causes flares or worsening of preexisting psoriasis.[51] Any clinical subtype of psoriasis can occur in patients with HIV but erythrodermic,[52] guttate, and inverse psoriasis are more common. This clinical subtype depends on the population studied. In HIV-positive patients, it is common for these subtypes to occur together in the same patient.[50]

Rupioid psoriasis (coin-shaped, hyperkeratotic crusted plaques) is another clinical form that can present in HIV-positive patients.[53] Sebopsoriasis is a term used when there are overlapping clinical features of psoriasis and seborrheic dermatitis. The lesions lack the typical psoriasiform scaling and are more crusted and exudative (**Fig. 15**). The seborrheic areas are usually involved and the treatment should include topical or systemic antifungals.[53] Dyspigmentation and a lack of erythema are common characteristics of psoriasis in pigmented skin.[54] Psoriatic arthritis is also

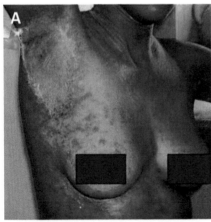 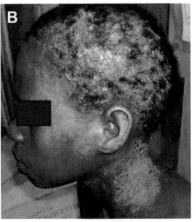

Fig. 13. Severe seborrheic dermatitis in HIV/AIDS. Note the extension of the dermatitis beyond the seborrheic areas.

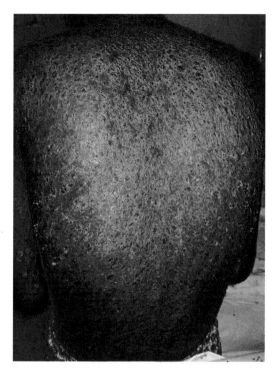

Fig. 14. Psoriasis in an HIV-positive patient. Widespread hyperpigmented plaques on the back. (*Courtesy of* Professor Anisa Mosam, PhD, University of KwaZulu-Natal, South Africa.)

more common and severe in the setting of HIV disease.[49,50]

In the setting of HIV/AIDS, psoriasis tends to be progressive and more resistant to treatment.[55] Treating psoriasis in HIV-positive patients is especially challenging due to the immunosuppressive effects of most of the systemic medications. Using these medications in already immunosuppressed patients can lead to serious complications.[50]

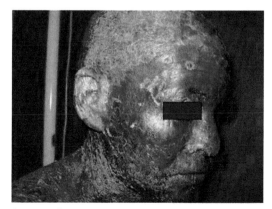

Fig. 15. Sebopsoriasis in an HIV-positive patient. Thick crusted plaques affecting the seborrheic areas of the face and scalp.

The general principle in treating HIV patients with psoriasis is to individualize the treatment according to a specific patient's needs. The severity of the psoriasis, other comorbidities, and the degree of immunosuppression due to the HIV should be kept in mind. The benefit-risk ratio for all treatment options should be carefully weighed and discussed with patients.[51] In 2010, a task force of the Medical Board of the National Psoriasis Foundation published a consensus document on the treatment of psoriasis in HIV disease.[51]

Their recommendations included the use of topical agents (calcipotriol [calcipotriene], corticosteroids, tazarotene, and a combination formulation of calcipotriol and betamethasone dipropionate) as the first-line treatment of mild to moderate disease. UV therapy (UV-B or psoralen–UV-A) and antiretrovirals should be used in moderate to severe psoriasis. Oral retinoids are second-line therapy for moderate to severe disease. In cases of more severe and refractory psoriasis, the immunosuppressants (cyclosporine, methotrexate, tumor necrosis factor [TNF]-α, inhibitors, and hydroxyurea) can be considered. When these drugs are used, however, it is important to carefully monitor patients for toxicities and side effects. All HIV patients with psoriasis need regular follow-up and careful monitoring for side effects. The management of patients with HIV and psoriasis is challenging and should preferably be in conjunction with an infectious diseases specialist.[51]

Reiter Syndrome

Reactive arthritis (Reiter syndrome) is characterized by the classic triad of urethritis, arthritis, and conjunctivitis.[56] As in HIV-negative patients, Reiter syndrome is usually triggered by preexisting gastrointestinal or urogenital infection. There is an association between Reiter syndrome and HIV, although reports in the literature vary. Some investigators report a prevalence of 4.6% in HIV-positive patients, which is 140 times higher than in the general population. This increase seems to be the highest, however, in HLA-B27–positive patients.[57] In a review of 3 large cohort studies, however, no association was found between HIV and Reiter syndrome.[58]

The mucocutaneous manifestations include thick hyperkeratotic plaques on the palms and soles (keratoderma blenorrhagicum), annular dermatitis on the glans penis (circinate balanitis), ulcerative vulvitis, oral lesions, and nail changes. The clinical picture in HIV-positive patients is usually more severe[56] and progressive in its course (**Fig. 16**).[55] In practice, the combination of mucocutaneous features, arthritis, and systemic

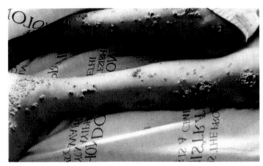

Fig. 16. Reiter syndrome in HIV/AIDS. Thick keratotic plaques on the lower legs.

symptoms can be difficult to distinguish from secondary syphilis.[59]

The treatment of the cutaneous lesions is the same as of HIV-negative patients and includes topical steroids and salicylic acid.[56] Immunosuppressive agents, as in the treatment of psoriasis, are generally not used. Acitretin could be used as an alternative systemic drug and improves skin and joint symptoms.[60] There are also reports of successful treatment with antiretroviral medication and TNF-α inhibitors.[61,62]

Pruritic Papular Eruption

Pruritic papular eruption (PPE) is a common cutaneous manifestation in patients with HIV infection. Although the cause is not clearly established, it is thought to be a hypersensitivity reaction to insect bites.[63] The histologic picture of PPE also confirms this theory.[63] The incidence of PPE varies between 12% and 46% depending on the geographic location.[64]

Clinically, PPE presents as extremely pruritic, symmetric, skin-colored to erythematous papules or pustules on the distal extremities (Fig. 17). With time, the eruption can become more widespread, affecting the trunk and face and making it difficult to distinguish from eosinophilic folliculitis.

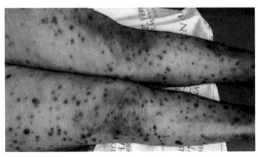

Fig. 17. PPE of HIV. Bilateral symmetric hyperpigmented papules and pustules on the legs. Note the extensive postlesional hyperpigmentation.

Bilateral, symmetric pruritic papules occurring for more than a month on the extremities are considered highly suggestive of PPE (79.2%).[64] Due to the pruritic nature of the disease, these papules become excoriated, secondarily infected, and prurigo nodularis–like.[65]

Hyperpigmentation is common in patients with pigmented skin and can lead to morbidity and stigmatization.[66] PPE occurs in patients with a low CD4+ count (<350 cells/μL) and usually in advanced HIV disease. Therefore, it could be considered a marker for immunosuppression and the initiation of antiretroviral medication in areas where resources are scarce.[64]

Symptomatic treatment with topical corticosteroids, emollients, and antihistamines are usually of limited value.[64] The cornerstone of treatment is the use of antiretroviral medication, often resulting in a dramatic improvement of symptoms. In contrast, recurrences may be associated with antiretroviral treatment failure.

It was, therefore, suggested that PPE can be used to monitor response to antiretroviral treatment in resource-poor areas.[67] In resistant cases, narrow-band UV-B phototherapy can also be considered a treatment option.[68]

Eosinophilic Folliculitis

Eosinophilic folliculitis (HIV-EF) is another pruritic eruption occurring in HIV-positive patients. HIV-EF is a unique disease entity and differs form classic EF (Ofuji disease), closely resembling PPE.[69] There are only quantitative differences in the histopathology and immunohistochemistry between PPE and EF. They can probably be considered, therefore, as different ends of a disease spectrum of hypersensitivity reactions in the setting of HIV disease.[70]

The exact incidence of HIV-EF is unknown, partly because the terms, PPE and HIV-EF, are used interchangeably in the literature. Follicular edematous papulovesicles or pustules mainly affecting the face, neck, and upper arms characterize this condition (Fig. 18). These papules are extremely pruritic and become secondary excoriated.[71] Postinflammatory hyperpigmentation is a major concern in patients with pigmented skin related to facial involvement in HIV-EF.

As in PPE, HIV-EF usually occurs in HIV patients with low CD4+ counts (<300 cells/μL). HIV-EF can also occur as part of the IRIS.[71]

The cause is debated, but a hypersensitivity reaction induced by various antigens in a dysregulated immune system is the most likely explanation.[69]

There is no specific treatment protocol for HIV-EF. Ketoconazole and griseofulvin have

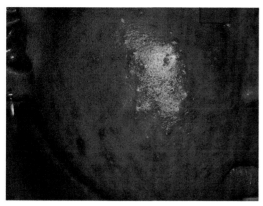

Fig. 18. HIV eosinophilic folliculitis. Numerous erythematous papules on the face. Excoriation, depigmentation, hyperpigmentation, and scarring are visible.

been used with positive results.[69] Oral antihistamines, metronidazole, itraconazole, prednisone, dapsone, ivermectin, and isotretinoin have also been used. Topical application of permethrin and 0.1% topical tacrolimus ointment may be beneficial. As for the treatment of PPE, the use of UV-B phototherapy can also be considered.[71] There is a definite improvement of HIV-EF with the use of antiretroviral therapy.[72]

Xerosis

Dry skin (xerosis) is a common finding in HIV-positive patients. In some studies, it is the most common skin manifestation (37.6%), even in patients on antiretroviral therapy.[33] It is also one of the major causes of pruritus in these patients.[73] It usually starts on the extremities[2] and becomes more widespread with time (**Fig. 19**).

Xerosis worsens with a decrease in the CD4+ count; therefore, it can be considered a marker for disease progression.[2] The cause is unknown, but changes in the blood flow and nutrient supply to the skin as well as diminished oil and sweat production in the skin could play a role.[2] The liberal use of emollients remains the cornerstone of treatment.

Photosensitivity Disorders

Photosensitivity is reported in approximately 5.4% of HIV-positive patients. It is also known that African Americans are 6.68 times more likely to develop photosensitivity.[74] The reason why patients with pigmented skin are disproportionately affected is unclear. Patients on antiretroviral medication are also more likely to develop photosensitivity.[74]

Although photosensitizing medications (trimethoprim-sulfamethoxazole, nonsteroidal inflammatory drugs, and antiretrovirals) can play a role in the pathogenesis, it is thought that HIV infection per se can cause photosensitivity.[75] Photosensitivity reactions usually manifest in patients with low CD4+ counts.[76]

Photosensitivity reactions observed in HIV patients include polymorphic light eruption, actinic prurigo, chronic actinic dermatitis, porphyria cutanea tarda, photosensitive granuloma annulare, and lichenoid photoeruptions.[75] Photosensitivity in HIV-positive patients has long been a well-recognized clinical entity.[74] The lesions are

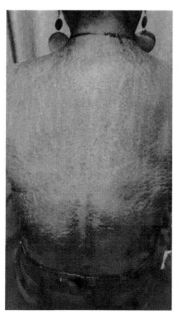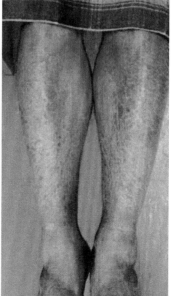

Fig. 19. Widespread xerosis in a HIV-positive patient, involving the back (*left*) and lower legs (*right*).

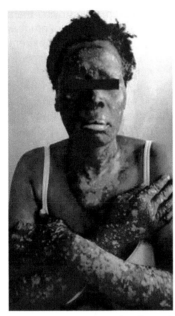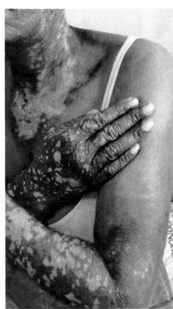

Fig. 20. Photodermatitis in HIV/AIDS. Note the sharp demarcation at covered areas. Dyspigmentation (hyperpigmentation and depigmentation) is clearly visible.

distributed in sun-exposed areas with a sharp demarcation at covered areas (**Fig. 20**). In severe cases, it can overflow to involve sun-protected skin and even become generalized. The clinical morphology varies and may resemble lichen planus or eczema.[74]

Hyperpigmentation is especially common in patients with pigmented skin. On the contrary, vitiligo-like depigmentation has also been described.[75] Treatment is difficult and sun protection and topical steroids are often used.[75]

SUMMARY

The introduction of antiretroviral medication has changed the epidemiology, morbidity, and mortality of HIV disease. Antiretrovirals have also altered the incidence of infective and inflammatory diseases affecting the skin. Nevertheless, cutaneous disorders due to HIV infection remain a major problem in HIV-infected patients. In patients with pigmented skin, HIV-associated dermatoses result in special challenges, particularly with regard to diagnosis and treatment. Due to the common problem of dyspigmentation caused by these conditions in pigmented skin, early diagnosis and effective treatment are of utmost importance. Clinicians should be aware of the differences in clinical presentation and the treatment options available. The influence of the HIV-associated dermatoses on a patient's quality of life should never be underestimated.

REFERENCES

1. Zancanaro PC, McGirt LY, Mamelak AJ, et al. Cutaneous manifestations of HIV in the era of highly active antiretroviral therapy: an institutional urban clinic experience. J Am Acad Dermatol 2006;54: 581–8.
2. Cedeno-Laurent F, Gómez-Flores M, Mendez N, et al. New insights into HIV-1-primary skin disorders. J Idaho Acad Sci 2011;14:1–11.
3. Amerson EH, Maurer TA. Dermatologic manifestations of HIV in Africa. Top HIV Med 2010;18:16–22.
4. Lupi O. Prevalence and risk factors for herpes simplex infection among patients at high risk for HIV infection in Brazil. Int J Dermatol 2011;50:709–13.
5. Draganova-Tacheva RA, Domsky S, Paralkar V, et al. Bacillary angiomatosis as an initial presentation in an HIV-positive Man. Clinl Microbiol Newsl 2009;31(19):150–2.
6. Grilo N, Modi D, Barrow P. Cutaneous bacillary angiomatosis: a marker of systemic disease in HIV. S Afr Med J 2009;99(4):220–1.
7. Muldoon EG, Mooka B, Reidy D, et al. Long-term neurological follow-up of HIV-positive patients diagnosed with syphilis. Int J STD AIDS 2012;23:676–8.
8. Zellen J, Augenbraun M. Syphilis in the HIV-infected patient: an update on epidemiology, diagnosis and management. Curr HIV/AIDS Rep 2004; 1:142–7.
9. Fleming DT, Wasserheit JN. From epidemiological synergy to public health policy and practice: the contribution of other sexually transmitted diseases

to sexual transmission of HIV infection. Sex Transm Infect 1999;75:3–17.

10. Zetola NM, Klausner JD. Syphilis and HIV infection: an update. Clin Infect Dis 2007;44:1222–8.

11. Knaute DF, Graf N, Lautenschlager S, et al. Serological response to treatment of syphilis according to disease stage and HIV status. Clin Infect Dis 2012;55:1615–22.

12. Wozniacka A, Schwartz RA, Sysa-Jedrzejowska A, et al. Lupus Vulgaris: report of two cases. Int J Dermatol 2005;44:299–301.

13. Padvamathy L, Ras LL, Ethirajan N, et al. Ulcerative Lupus Vulgaris of face: an uncommon presentation in India. Indian J Tuberc 2007;54:52–4.

14. Libraty DH, Byrd TF. Cutaneous miliary tuberculosis in the AIDS era: case report and review. Clin Infect Dis 1996;23:706–10.

15. Daikos GL, Uttamchandani RB, Tuda C, et al. Disseminated miliary tuberculosis of the skin in patients with AIDS: report of four cases. Clin Infect Dis 1998;27:205–8.

16. Regnier S, Ouagari Z, Perez L, et al. Cutaneous Miliary resistant tuberculosis in a patient infected with human immunodeficiency virus: case report and literature review. Clin Exp Dermatol 2009;34: e690–2.

17. Fernandes C, Maltez F, Lourenco S, et al. Papulonecrotic tuberculid in a human immunodeficiency virus type-1 patient with multidrug- resistant tuberculosis. J Eur Acad Dermatol Venereol 2004;18:369–94.

18. Akhras V, McCarthy G. Papulonecrotic tuberculid in an HIV-positive patient. Int J STD AIDS 2007; 18:643–4.

19. Clayton YM. Superficial fungal infections. In: Harper J, Orange A, Prose N, editors. Textbook of pediatric dermatology. London: Blackwell Science; 2002. p. 447–72.

20. Nweze EI. Dermatophytoses in Western Africa: a review. Pak J Biol Sci 2010;13(3):649–56.

21. Petmy JL, Lando AJ, Kaptue L, et al. Superficial mycoses and HIV infection in Yaounde. J Eur Acad Dermatol Venereol 2004;18:301–4.

22. Aly R, Berger T. Common superficial fungal infections in patients with AIDS. Clin Infect Dis 1996; 22(Suppl 2):S128–32.

23. Elmets CA. Management of common superficial fungal infections in patients with AIDS. J Am Acad Dermatol 1994;31:S60–3.

24. Durden FM, Elewski B. Fungal infections in HIV-Infected patients. Semin Cutan Med Surg 1997; 16(3):200–12.

25. Ramos-e-Silva M, Lima CM, Schechtman RC, et al. Systemic mycoses in immunodepressed patients (AIDS). Clin Dermatol 2012;30:616–27.

26. Portu JJ, Santamaria JM, Zubero Z, et al. Atypical scabies in HIV-positive patients. J Am Acad Dermatol 1996;34:915–7.

27. Jessurun J, Romo-Garcia J, Lopez-Denis O, et al. Crusted scabies in a patient with the acquired immunodeficiency syndrome. Virchows Arch A Pathol Anat Histopathol 1990;415:461–3.

28. Sampaio AL, Mameri AC, Vargas TJ, et al. Seborrhoeic dermatitis. An Bras Dermatol 2011;86: 1061–74.

29. Stefanaki I, Katsambas A. Therapeutic update on seborrhoeic dermatitis. Skin Therapy Lett 2010; 15:1–4.

30. Palamaras I, Kyriakis KP, Stavrianeas NG. Seborrhoeic dermatitis: lifetime detection rates. J Eur Acad Dermatol Venereol 2012;26:524–6.

31. Mathes BM, Douglass MC. Seborrhoeic dermatitis in patients with acquired immunodeficiency syndrome. J Am Acad Dermatol 1985;13:947–51.

32. Soeprono FF, Schinella RA, Cockerell CJ, et al. Seborrhoeic-like dermatitis of acquired immunodeficiency syndrome. A clinicopathologic study. J Am Acad Dermatol 1986;14(2 Part 1):242–8.

33. Blanes M, Belinchón I, Merino E, et al. Current prevalence and characteristics of dermatoses associated with human immunodeficiency virus infection. Actas Dermosifiliogr 2010;101(8):702–9.

34. Wikler JR, Nieboer C, Willemze R. Quantitative skin cultures of Pityrosporum yeasts in patients seropositive for the humanimmunodeficiency virus with and without seborrhoeic dermatitis. J Am Acad Dermatol 1992;27:37–9.

35. Eisenstat BA, Wormser GP. Seborrhoeic dematitis and butterfly rash in AIDS [letter]. N Engl J Med 1984;189:311.

36. Rincón S, Celis A, Sopó L, et al. Malassezia yeast species isolated from patients with dermatologic lesions. Biomedica 2005;25:189–95.

37. Bergbrant IM, Johansson S, Robbins D, et al. An immunological study in patients with seborrhoeic dermatitis. Clin Exp Dermatol 1991;16:331–8.

38. Marino CT, McDonald E, Romano JF. Seborrhoeic dermatitis in acquired immunodeficiency syndrome. Cutis 1991;50:217–8.

39. Alessi E, Cusini M, Zerboni R. Mucocutaneous manifestations in patients infected with human immunodeficiency virus. J Am Acad Dermatol 1988; 19(2 Part 1):290–7.

40. Matis WL, Triana A, Shapiro R, et al. Dermatologic findings associated with human immunodeficiency virus infection. J Am Acad Dermatol 1987;17: 46–51.

41. Senaldi G, Di Perri G, Di Silverio A, et al. Seborrhoeic dermatitis:an early manifestation in AIDS [letter]. Clin Exp Dermatol 1987;12:72–3.

42. Vidal C, Girard PM, Dompmartin D, et al. Seborrhoeic dermatitis and HIV infection: qualitative analysis of skin surface lipids in men seropositive and seronegative for HIV. J Am Acad Dermatol 1990;23(6 Part 1):1106–10.

43. Mahe A, Simon F, Coulibaly S. Predictive value of seborrhoeic dermatitis and other common dermatoses for HIV infection in Bamako, Mali. J Am Acad Dermatol 1988;38:1084–6.

44. Puig L, Fernandez-Figueras T, Ferrandiz C, et al. Epidermal expression of 65 and 72 kD heat shock proteins in psoriasis and AIDS-associated psoriasiform dermatitis. J Am Acad Dermatol 1995;33:985–9.

45. Dann FJ, Tabibian P. Cutaneous diseases in human immunodeficiency virus-infected patients referred to the UCLA Immunosuppression Skin Clinic: reasons for referral and management of select diseases. Cutis 1995;55:85–8.

46. Ford GP, Farr PM, Ive FA, et al. The response of seborrhoeic dermatitis to ketoconazole. Br J Dermatol 1984;111:603–9.

47. Buchness MR. Treatment of skin diseases in HIV-infected patients. Dermatol Clin 1995;13:231–8.

48. Ortonne JP, Lacour JP, Vitetta A, et al. Comparative study of ketoconazole 2% foaming gel and betamethasone dipropionate 0.05% lotion in the treatment of seborrhoeic dermatitis in adults. Dermatology 1992;184:275–80.

49. Mallon E, Bunker CB. HIV-associated psoriasis. AIDS Patient Care STDS 2000;14:239–46.

50. Montazeri A, Kanitakis J, Bazex J. Psoriasis and HIV infection. Int J Dermatol 1996;35:475–9.

51. Menon K, Van Voorhees AS, Bebo BF, et al. Psoriasis in patients with HIV infection: from the Medical Board of the National Psoriasis Foundation. J Am Acad Dermatol 2010;62:291–9.

52. Morar N, Dlova N, Gupta AK, et al. Erythroderma: a comparison between HIV positive and negative patients. Int J Dermatol 1999;38:895–900.

53. Morar N, Willis-Owen SA, Maurer T, et al. HIV-associated psoriasis: pathogenesis, clinical features, and management. Lancet Infect Dis 2010;10:470–8.

54. McMichael AJ, Vachiramon V, Guzmán-Sánchez DA, et al. Psoriasis in African-Americans: a caregivers' survey. J Drugs Dermatol 2012;1(4):478–82.

55. Duvic M, Johnson IM, Rapini RE, et al. Acquired immunodeficiency syndrome-associated Psoriasis and Reiter's syndrome. Arch Dermatol 1987;123:1622–32.

56. Wu IB, Schwartz RA. Reiter's syndrome: the classic triad and more. J Am Acad Dermatol 2008;59:113–21.

57. Winchester R, Brancato L, Itescu S, et al. Implications from the occurrence of Reiter's syndrome and related disorders in association with advanced HIV infection. Scand J Rheumatol Suppl 1988;74:89–93.

58. Clark MR, Solinger AM, Hochberg MC. Human immunodeficiency virus infection is not associated with Reiter's syndrome: data from three large cohort studies. Rheum Dis Clin North Am 1992;18:267–76.

59. Kishimoto M, Lee MJ, Mor A, et al. Syphilis mimicking Reiter's syndrome in an HIV-positive patient. Am J Med Sci 2006;332(2):90–2.

60. Blanche P. Acitretin and AIDS-related Reiter's disease. Clin Exp Rheumatol 1999;17:105–6.

61. McGonagle D, Reade S, Marzo-Ortega H, et al. Human immunodeficiency virus associated spondyloarthropathy: pathogenic insights based on imaging findings and response to highly active antiretroviral treatment. Ann Rheum Dis 2001;60:696–8.

62. Gaylis N. Infliximab in the treatment of an HIV positive patient with Reiter's syndrome. J Rheumatol 2003;30:407–11.

63. Resnick JS Jr, Van Beek M, Furmanski L, et al. Etiology of pruritic papular eruption with HIV infection in Uganda. JAMA 2004;292:2614–21.

64. Farsani TT, Kore S, Nadol P, et al. Etiology and risk factors associated with a pruritic papular eruption in people living with HIV in India. J International AIDS Society 2013;16:1–6.

65. Hevia O, Jimenez-Acosta F, Ceballos P, et al. Pruritic papular eruption of the acquired. J Am Acad Dermatol 1991;24:231–5.

66. Muyinda H, Seeley J, Pickerine H, et al. Social aspects of AIDS-related stigma in rural Uganda. Health Place 1997;3:143–7.

67. Castelnuovo B, Byakwaga H, Menten J, et al. Can response of a pruritic papular eruption to antiretroviral therapy be used as a clinical parameter to monitor virological outcome? AIDS 2008;22:269–73.

68. Bellavista S, D'Antuono A, Infusino SD, et al. Pruritic papular eruption in HIV: a case successfully treated with NB-UVB. Dermatol Ther 2013;26(2):173–5.

69. Nervi SJ, Schwartz RA, Dmochowski M. Eosinophilic pustular folliculitis: a 40 year retrospect. J Am Acad Dermatol 2006;55:285–9.

70. Afonso JP, Tomimori J, Michalany NS, et al. Pruritic papular eruption and eosinophilic folliculitis associated with human immunodeficiency virus (HIV) infection: a histopathological and immunohistochemical comparative study. J Am Acad Dermatol 2012;67:269–75.

71. Eisman S. Pruritic papular eruption in HIV. Dermatol Clin 2006;24:449–57.

72. Rajendran PM, Dolev JC, Heaphy MR Jr, et al. Eosinophilic folliculitis: before and after the introduction of antiretroviral therapy. Arch Dermatol 2005;141:1227–31.

73. Blanes M, Belinchón I, Portilla J, et al. Pruritus in HIV-infected patients in the era of combination antiretroviral therapy: a study of its prevalence and causes. Int J STD AIDS 2012;23(4):255–7.

74. Bilu D, Mamelak AJ, Nguyen RH, et al. Clinical and epidemiologic characterization of photosensitivity in HIV-positive individuals. Photodermatol Photoimmunol Photomed 2004;20:175–83.

75. Philips RC, Motaparthi K, Krishnan B, et al. HIV photodermatitis presenting with widespread vitiligo-like depigmentation. Dermatol Online J 2012;18(1):6. Available at: http://escholarship.org/uc/item/74h8t36w. Accessed September 20, 2013.

76. Berger TG, Dhar A. Lichenoid photoeruptions in human immunodeficiency virus infection. Arch Dermatol 1994;130(5):609–13.

Clinical Presentations of Severe Cutaneous Drug Reactions in HIV-Infected Africans

Rannakoe J. Lehloenya, BSc, MBChB, FCDerm(SA)[a],*,
Mahlatse Kgokolo, BPharm, MBChB, MMed, FCDerm(SA)[b]

KEYWORDS

• HIV • Drug eruptions • Africans • Clinical characteristics • Review

KEY POINTS

• The incidence of cutaneous adverse drug reactions (CADRs) is high in HIV-infected persons; however, there are large gaps in knowledge about several aspects of HIV-associated CADRs in Africa, which carries the biggest burden of the disease.
• Gaps include epidemiology, pathomechanisms, pharmacogenetics, and management strategies.
• Population studies are needed to better inform policymakers and clinicians on the optimal management of HIV-associated CADRs.
• Some of these studies can be extrapolated from data arising elsewhere with reasonable accuracy whereas others, like pharmacogenetics, have to be done in African populations in Africa.

INTRODUCTION

Sub-Saharan Africa is the epicenter of the HIV pandemic, accounting for 68% of the global burden of the disease. The disease has changed the epidemiology and the profile of dermatology practice in Africa, with higher incidences of inflammatory dermatoses, infections, and drug eruptions compared to the general population.[1–6] Although highly active antiretroviral therapy (HAART) and effective treatments for HIV-associated opportunistic infections have had a dramatic impact on reducing HIV-related morbidity and mortality, they are associated with many complications, including drug-related toxicities, drug interactions, and immune reconstitution inflammatory syndrome (IRIS). It is estimated that drug hypersensitivity reactions, related to a wide spectrum of drugs, are 2 to 100 times more common in HIV-infected persons, with the actual figure probably somewhere in-between the 2 extremes.[7–10]

There are many classifications used for adverse drug reactions, and the simplest divides them into 2 types, depending on whether they are predictable and dose dependent (type A) or unpredictable and dose independent (type B).[11,12] This review focuses on the latter, which accounts for 15% to 20% of all adverse drug reactions. The epidemiology and the clinical spectrum of HIV-associated type B CADRs in African populations, excluding IgE-mediated reactions, are discussed.

EPIDEMIOLOGY OF HIV-ASSOCIATED CADRS IN AFRICA

Accurate data on the incidence of HIV-associated CADRs worldwide, particularly in Africa, are limited by lack of population-based studies, inconsistency in the design of published studies, inaccurate reporting, and limitations in case definitions and disease severity grading.[13,14] This applies to both CADRs in general and the

[a] Division of Dermatology, Department of Medicine, University of Cape Town, Anzio Road, Observatory, Cape Town, South Africa 7925; [b] Department of Dermatology, University of Pretoria, and Steve Biko Hospital, Dr Savage Street, Pretoria, South Africa 0001
* Corresponding author. Ward G23, New Groote Schuur Hospital, Anzio Road, Observatory 7925, South Africa.
E-mail address: rannakoe.lehloenya@uct.ac.za

Dermatol Clin 32 (2014) 227–235
http://dx.doi.org/10.1016/j.det.2013.11.004

individual phenotypes of drug reactions. As such, patient-related outcomes and the overall impact on the health care system of HIV-associated CADRs are largely unknown.

The limited available data from Africa in hospitalized patients and outpatient clinics suggest that the incidence is significantly higher than in the general population. Drug-induced erythroderma in HIV-infected patients ranged from 20% of all erythrodermas in a Nigerian study to 41% at a teaching hospital in Durban, South Africa.[15–17] Up to 80% of the cases presenting with Stevens-Johnson syndrome (SJS) and toxic epidermal necrolysis (TEN) at 2 tertiary hospitals in Cape Town, South Africa, were HIV infected.[18,19]

PHARMACOGENETICS OF CADRS IN AFRICA

CADRs are associated with specific HLA subtypes in some populations. Good examples are the Han Chinese and many populations in Southeast Asia where SJS and TEN secondary to carbamezapine has an association with HLA-B*1502 in almost all cases; and in both the Han Chinese and whites there is an association between HLA-B*5801 and allopurinol-induced SJS and TEN.[20–22] Abacavir-induced hypersensitivity syndrome is strongly associated with HLA-B*5701 during treatment of HIV infection, and prospective studies have shown that HLA-B*5701 screening reduces the incidence of hypersensitivity reactions. This association seems generalizable across racial groups in Asia, Europe, and the Unites States.[23,24] In the only large study to date performed in Africa, however, HLA-B*5701 was not significantly associated with clinically diagnosed abacavir hypersensitivity reaction in patients of African race from Uganda.[25] Pharmacogenetics of CADRs are drug specific and population specific, and more studies in Africa are needed to characterize the association between genetic predisposition and HIV-associated CADRs as the world moves toward individualized medical therapies and diagnostics.

TYPES OF CADRS

Types of HIV-associated CADRs range from mild transient eruptions to severe life-threatening forms. The clinical features can either be confined to the skin or be part of a multisystem disorder. They include morbiliform drug eruptions, SJS and TEN, and drug reaction with eosinophilia and systemic symptoms (DRESS) syndrome. There are other types of CADRs, however, that do not seem to be higher in HIV-infected persons compared with the general population. These include urticaria, lichenoid drug eruptions, fixed drug eruption (FDEs), acute generalized exanthematous pustulosis, photodermatitis, and cutaneous vasculitis.[1]

A specific drug is generally not associated with a specific phenotype of CADR and a specific type of CADR can be due to any drug.[13] A case in point is nevirapine, which is strongly associated with SJS and TEN, morbilliform eruptions, and DRESS in both adults and children.[26–29] There are, however, certain drugs that are more commonly associated with some types of CADRs. A good historical example is thioacetazone, which was strongly associated with SJS and TEN in tuberculosis and HIV coinfected patients, leading to the World Health Organization recommending avoidance of the drug with subsequent decline of its use worldwide.[30]

Morbiliform Drug Eruptions

Morbilliform (measles-like) drug eruptions, also referred to as maculopapular rash, account for 95% of all cases of CADRs.[31] The rash presents as centrifugally spreading erythematous macules and papules that sometimes become confluent. Morbilliform drug eruptions are usually self-limiting and treatment interruption is not necessary.[32] They are differentiated from DRESS by a lack of systemic involvement and from SJS and TEN by absence of epidermal necrosis and mucositis. At the initial presentation, however, these differences may not be obvious and attending clinicians should be aware of the possibility of progression to more severe disease **Fig. 1**.[33–35]

Drug Rash with Eosinophilia and Systemic Symptoms

DRESS syndrome or drug hypersensitivity syndrome is characterized by prodromal symptoms of pruritus and pyrexia followed by fever, edema,

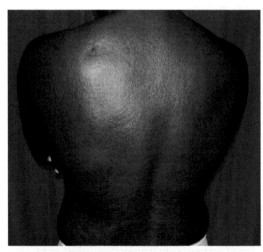

Fig. 1. Morbilliform eruption without systemic features in an HIV-infected woman.

lymphadenopathy, leukocyte abnormalities (leucocytosis, eosinophilia, and/or atypical lymphocytosis), hepatitis, and a long latency period (>3 weeks). Rarely nephritis, pancreatitis, pneumonitis, and myocarditis are the other systemic features. The rash presents as a ubiquitous exanthema that may be urticarial, maculopapular, vesicular, pustular, purpuric, targetoid, or erythrodermic.[36,37] Visceral involvement differentiates DRESS syndrome from the other eruptions that are not drug related, including viral exanthemata, inflammatory conditions, and HIV-associated atypical cutaneous lymphoproliferative disorders. Because the clinical features can be identical, irrespective of the cause, these have to be excluded **Fig. 2**.[38–42] There are few data suggesting that DRESS syndrome is more common in persons with African ancestry and it is well established that in Africa the incidence is higher in HIV-infected persons.[15,16,33,41]

As in all types of CADRs, early withdrawal of the offending drug(s) improves outcomes in DRESS. In mild disease, characterized amongst others by transaminitis less than 5 times the upper limit of normal, absence of pneumonitis, hemophagocytosis or pancreatitis, topical steroids with emmolients, and antihistamines are usually effective. In severe disease, systemic steroids are warranted.[43] Based on the authors' experience, in most cases, the rash is mild and responds to topical steroids. The severity of the rash, however, is not always proportional to the severity of the systemic involvement and the abnormal laboratory parameters may persist for several days to several months after withdrawal of the offending drug.

The most common causes of death in DRESS syndrome are liver failure and sepsis.[44] DRESS syndrome–associated mortality in HIV is unknown, but in the general population it is estimated to be between 3.7% and 10%.[28,36,44,45] DRESS syndrome is associated with long-term sequelae and in darker skin these include persistent postinflammatory hyperpigmentation, chronic exfoliative dermatitis, cutaneous scarring, and nail changes. There are emerging reports of patients developing autoimmune diseases after DRESS syndrome.[46] These reports need further validation in larger prospective studies.

Stevens-Johnson Syndrome and Toxic Epidermal Necrolysis

SJS and TEN are considered on the spectrum of the same disease. They are delineated by percentage body surface area of epidermal necrosis and stripping. In SJS there is less than 10% of epidermal detachment and in TEN there is greater than 30%. SJS/TEN overlap lies between these 2 extremes. Rarely, systemic features are present. The early clinical features, often confused with upper respiratory tract infection, include fever, malaise, cough, stinging eyes, and a sore throat. This is followed by rapid progression to epidermal necrosis and detachment, mucositis, and painful blistering of the palms and soles **Fig. 3**. The incidence of SJS and TEN is as high as 1 to 2 per 1000 individuals in HIV-infected cohorts, much higher than in the general population.[47] Of all CADRs, TEN has the highest mortality, of up to 35%, as reported in a South African population.[48] In most cases, mortality is due to skin and mucosal failure, resulting in bacterial systemic infections.[49] It is controversial whether systemic steroids and intravenous immunoglobulins are beneficial in SJS and TEN but there is a general consensus

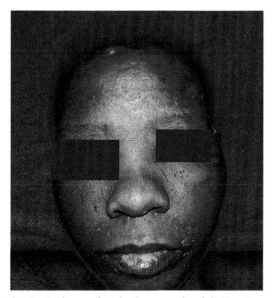

Fig. 2. Erythema, facial edema, and exfoliation in a patient with DRESS syndrome.

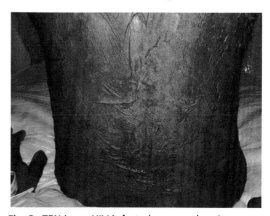

Fig. 3. TEN in an HIV-infected woman showing a positive Nikolsky sign and small areas of early epidermal denudation.

that antibiotics should only be used in the presence of clinical and/or microbiological features of an infection. Supportive therapy is the mainstay of treatment paired with a multidisciplinary approach.[50–52]

SJS and TEN are debilitating diseases with long-term sequelae of varying severity. These range from moderate dry eye syndrome to blindness; esophageal strictures; hematocolpos, vulvovaginal synechiae, and fibrosis; heterotrophic calcifications; dyspigmentation; and hypertrophic scars **Fig. 4**.[27,53–57] The authors have recently shown a higher incidence of depression and anxiety in a predominantly HIV-infected cohort of SJS and TEN cases 6 weeks after the resolution of acute symptoms. Considering the high incidence of SJS and TEN in HIV-infected people, there are few studies documenting and advising on the management of long-term sequelae in this population.

Lichenoid Drug Reactions

Lichenoid drug reactions (LDRs) are characterized by violaceous macules and plaques on the skin and are characteristic white lace pattern, called Wickham striae, in the mucosae. The authors have encountered a few cases of LDRs in HIV-infected persons, mainly related to antituberculosis drugs. The incidence of LDRs in HIV does not seem higher than in the general population.[58] The challenge in LDRs is the lack of acute markers, insidious onset of the rash, wide variation in the intervals between drug initiation, and a clinically detectable rash. All these make it difficult to establish a temporal relationship with the offending drug and ascribe causality. In cases of polypharmacy with limited number of effective drugs, as is the case in the treatment of AIDS and tuberculosis, this creates a major therapeutic conundrum. In tuberculosis-associated LDRs, the authors' experience has shown that sometimes the benefits of continuing therapy outweigh the risks of ongoing CADRs and treatment is carried through to completion of the course. This results in increasing and persistent hyperpigmentation, focal areas of depigmentation, hyperkeratosis, and painful fissuring of the skin, all of which seem more severe in darker African skin **Fig. 5**.

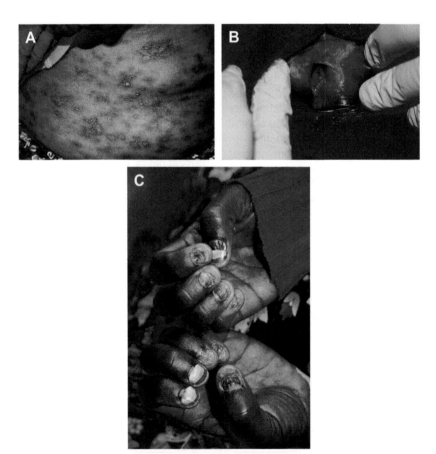

Fig. 4. (*A*) Scarring, hyperpigmentation, and milia after SJS. (*B*) Scarring of the labia minora after genital involvement in SJS. (*C*) Pterygium of the nail in a patient with SJS.

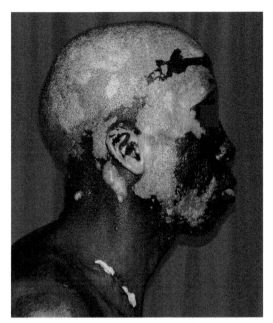

Fig. 5. Lichenoid drug eruption with depigmentation in an HIV-infected man on treatment of a second episode of tuberculosis with Rifafour, a combination drug of rifampicin, isoniazid, pyrazinamide, and ethambutol. The rash initially developed during the first course of tuberculosis treatment and resulted in areas of depigmentation and hyperpigmentation. This picture shows recurrence with violaceous patches within the depigmented areas from the first episode.

Potent topical steroids and phototherapy can be used to control the eruption until the course is completed.[13,58]

Fixed Drug Eruptions

FDEs presents as a solitary or numerous itchy, round, well-circumscribed macules that resolve with persistent hyperpigmentation. They recur at exactly the same sites on re-exposure to the offending drug, sometimes with new lesions erupting elsewhere.[59] FDEs are uncommon and there is no evidence of them associated with HIV infection.[60] There are reports, however, of FDEs secondary to protease inhibitors used for treatment of HIV. The FDEs appeared at initiation of therapy and resolved despite continuing therapeutic doses of the drugs with further recurrence when treatment was stopped and then reinitiated.[61] These few data suggest that if there are limited therapeutic options and the FDE is localized and nonbullous, there is room for continuation of therapy. This needs to be substantiated, however, in larger series of patients.

Efavirenz-associated CADRs

The authors have recently described photo-distribution and annular erythema as features of efavirenz-associated CADRs without significant systemic involvement. The reactions occurred when the drug was a constituent of a fixed-dose once-a-day combination antiretroviral drugs and as part of HAART comprising separate agents **Fig. 6**.[62,63] What is not yet clear is whether the reactions to efavirenz are truly mild and transient or if they represent early signs of severe CADRs warranting interruption or termination of therapy. With the increasing use of efavirenz-containing fixed-dose regimen in sub-Saharan Africa because of their ease of use and improvement in patient compliance, more of these reactions are likely to be encountered and more studies needed to characterize them and develop appropriate management strategies.[63]

SPECIAL CONSIDERATIONS IN HIV-ASSOCIATED CADRS
Multiple Drug Hypersensitivity Reactions

Multiple drug hypersensitivity (MDH) is a predilection to react to different chemically and structurally

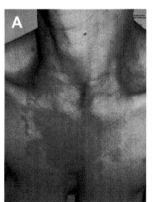
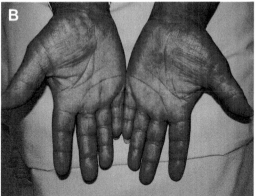

Fig. 6. (A) Annular erythema of the V of the neck and (B) tender indurated palmar erythema in a patient recently started on Odimune, a once-daily combination antiretroviral drug comprising efavirenz, tenofovir, and emtricitabine.

unrelated drugs that are metabolized through different pathways, with no evidence of cross-reactivity.[64] The authors have recently shown a high incidence of MDH in tuberculosis-HIV coinfected African patients due to first- and second-line antituberculosis drugs. Since the publication of the report, the authors have encountered an increasing number of similar reactions. The spectrum of CADRs included DRESS, SJS and TEN, and anaphylactoid reactions, the latter sometimes associated with severe neurologic sequelae.[65] MDH has been reported for many classes of drugs and the authors' findings suggest that the incidence is higher in HIV-infected persons. This is possibly due to the heightened immune stimulation in these patients, facilitating an enhanced response to multiple drugs in susceptible individuals. Clinicians should be aware of MDH, which may confuse the clinical picture if alternative therapies are introduced during an evolving CADR to the initial therapy. Further studies are needed to establish the pathogenesis, epidemiology, and clinical features of HIV-associated MDH.

Immune Reconstitution Inflammatory Syndrome

Initiation of HAART in HIV-infected persons leads to the restoration of host immunity and may be associated with the development of IRIS. The overlapping temporal and clinical characteristics of IRIS and CADRs often lead to clinical and diagnostic uncertainty. In addition, some investigators suggest that a CADR, in particular DRESS, is itself a form of IRIS.[66] Clinicians in high HIV-burden settings should thus exclude IRIS to avoid inappropriate interruption or termination of HAART.[67]

Systemic Reactions to Patch Tests and Skin Prick Tests

The authors recently reported a case of recurring DRESS secondary to re-exposure to rifampicin as a patch test. This case is part of an ongoing study of rechallenge with first-line drugs after severe CADRs to antituberculosis drugs.[68] Since this report, the authors have encountered more cases of systemic reactions to patch and prick tests on re-exposure to the offending drug without a localized reaction at the site of the test. The authors hypothesize that this is a result of HIV-associated immune dysregulation, which lowers the threshold of T cell activation, coupled with persistent stimulation of CD8[+] T cells.[69] The mechanism involved in this type of reaction may explain the high incidence of CADRs in HIV-infected people and needs further investigations.

CADRs in Pregnancy

In Africa, nevirapine is still widely used for prevention of mother-to-child transmission in HIV-infected pregnant women and it is a well-established cause of CADRs. A systematic review by Bera and colleagues[70] showed that pregnancy itself might be an additional risk factor for nevirapine-associated drug reactions. A recent case-control study by the authors at Groote Schuur Hospital in Cape Town, South Africa, found pregnancy associated with CADRs on univariate analysis; however, this was lost on multivariate analysis when compared with men.[71] Because of these side effects, concerns are being raised about the continuing use of nevirapine in HIV. There are no large studies, to the authors' knowledge, reporting on the effect of CADRs on pregnancy outcomes. In practice, the authors have encountered few intrauterine fetal deaths associated with SJS/TEN. It is not clear, however, whether these are related to CADRs or if the incidence is higher than in the general population and further studies are required to answer these questions.

SJS and TEN-associated Anxiety and Depression

There is ample and consistent evidence that depression is independently associated with poor adherence to medication, even in patients with no background of severe drug reactions.[72] In HIV-infected persons, continuation and/or reinitiation of HAART and therapy for opportunistic infections is imperative, even in the face of severe CADRs. There are few data on the impact of CADRs, however, on depression and compliance in HIV-infected persons. In a recent study the authors conducted in Cape Town of 32 consecutive cases of SJS/TEN, there was persistent anxiety and depression after SJS/TEN. TEN, the more severe form of SJS/TEN was significantly associated with more severe depression and anxiety.[73] These findings, if further substantiated in more studies, have major implications not only for long-term mental status of this population but also for compliance with medication.

SUMMARY

The incidence of CADRs is high in HIV-infected persons. There are large gaps in the knowledge, however, about several aspects of HIV-associated CADRs in Africa, which carries the biggest burden of the disease. These include gaps in epidemiology, pathomechanisms, pharmacogenetics, and management strategies.

Population studies are needed to better inform policymakers and clinicians on the optimal management of HIV-associated CADRs. Some of these can be extrapolated from data arising elsewhere with reasonable accuracy whereas others, like pharmacogenetics, have to be done in African populations in Africa.

REFERENCES

1. Ukonu AB, Eze EU. Pattern of skin diseases at university of Benin teaching hospital, Benin city, Edo State, South-South Nigeria: a 12 month prospective study. Glob J Health Sci 2012;4:148–57.
2. Joint United Nations Programme on AIDS: UNAIDS World AIDS Day Report 2011. Geneva: UNAIDS; 2011. Edition 2011.
3. Konare HD, Cisse IA, Oumar AA, et al. Cutaneous drug eruption at hospital in Bamako. Mali Med 2012;27:57–61 [in French].
4. Khambaty MM, Hsu SS. Dermatology of the patient with HIV. Emerg Med Clin North Am 2010;28:355–68 [Table of Contents].
5. Mosam A, Irusen EM, Kagoro H, et al. The impact of human immunodeficiency virus/acquired immunodeficiency syndrome (HIV/AIDS) on skin disease in KwaZulu-Natal, South Africa. Int J Dermatol 2004;43:782–3.
6. Punyaratabandhu P, Prasithsirikul W, Jirachanakul P. Skin manifestation of Thai HIV infected patients in HAART era. J Med Assoc Thai 2012;95:497–504.
7. Fritsch PO, Sidoroff A. Drug-induced Stevens-Johnson syndrome/toxic epidermal necrolysis. Am J Clin Dermatol 2000;1:349–60.
8. Coopman SA, Johnson RA, Platt R, et al. Cutaneous disease and drug reactions in HIV infection. N Engl J Med 1993;328:1670–4.
9. Kuaban C, Bercion R, Koula-Shiro S. Current HIV seroprevalence rate and incidence of adverse skin reactions in adults with pulmonary tuberculosis receiving thiacetazone-free antituberculosis treatment in Yaounde, Cameroon. Cent Afr J Med 1998;44:34–7.
10. Marks DJ, Dheda K, Dawson R, et al. Adverse events to antituberculosis therapy: influence of HIV and antiretroviral drugs. Int J STD AIDS 2009; 20:339–45.
11. Edwards IR, Aronson JK. Adverse drug reactions: definitions, diagnosis, and management. Lancet 2000;356:1255–9.
12. Aronson JK, Ferner RE. Joining the DoTS: new approach to classifying adverse drug reactions. BMJ 2003;327:1222–5.
13. Lehloenya RJ, Dheda K. Cutaneous adverse drug reactions to anti-tuberculosis drugs: state of the art and into the future. Expert Rev Anti Infect Ther 2012;10:475–86.
14. Todd G. Adverse cutaneous drug eruptions and HIV: a clinician's global perspective. Dermatol Clin 2006;24:459–72, vi.
15. Salami TA, Enahoro Oziegbe O, Omeife H. Exfoliative dermatitis: patterns of clinical presentation in a tropical rural and suburban dermatology practice in Nigeria. Int J Dermatol 2012;51: 1086–9.
16. Morar N, Dlova N, Gupta AK, et al. Erythroderma: a comparison between HIV positive and negative patients. Int J Dermatol 1999;38:895–900.
17. Salami TA, Asalu AF, Samuel SO. Prevalence of cutaneous drug eruptions in adult Nigerians with HIV/AIDS. Niger Postgrad Med J 2010;17:160–3.
18. Lehloenya RJ, Todd G, Badri M, et al. Outcomes of reintroducing anti-tuberculosis drugs following cutaneous adverse drug reactions. Int J Tuberc Lung Dis 2011;15:1649–57.
19. Kannenberg SM, Jordaan HF, Koegelenberg CF, et al. Toxic epidermal necrolysis and Stevens-Johnson syndrome in South Africa: a 3-year prospective study. QJM 2012;105:839–46.
20. Chung WH, Hung SI, Hong HS, et al. Medical genetics: a marker for Stevens-Johnson syndrome. Nature 2004;428:486.
21. Hung SI, Chung WH, Liou LB, et al. HLA-B*5801 allele as a genetic marker for severe cutaneous adverse reactions caused by allopurinol. Proc Natl Acad Sci U S A 2005;102:4134–9.
22. Wei CY, Ko TM, Shen CY, et al. A recent update of pharmacogenomics in drug-induced severe skin reactions. Drug Metab Pharmacokinet 2012;27: 132–41.
23. Mallal S, Phillips E, Carosi G, et al. HLA-B*5701 screening for hypersensitivity to abacavir. N Engl J Med 2008;358:568–79.
24. Saag M, Balu R, Phillips E, et al. High sensitivity of human leukocyte antigen-b*5701 as a marker for immunologically confirmed abacavir hypersensitivity in white and black patients. Clin Infect Dis 2008; 46:1111–8.
25. Munderi P, Snowden WB, Walker AS, et al. Distribution of HLA-B alleles in a Ugandan HIV-infected adult population: NORA pharmacogenetic substudy of DART. Trop Med Int Health 2011;16: 200–4.
26. Minniear TD, Zeh C, Polle N, et al. Rash, hepatotoxicity and hyperbilirubinemia among Kenyan infants born to HIV-infected women receiving triple-antiretroviral drugs for the prevention of mother-to-child HIV transmission. Pediatr Infect Dis J 2012;31:1155–7.
27. Saka B, Kombate K, Mouhari-Toure A, et al. Stevens-Johnson syndrome and toxic epidermal necrolysis in a teaching hospital in Lome, Togo: retrospective study of 89 cases. Med Trop (Mars) 2010;70:255–8 [in French].

28. Wongkitisophon P, Chanprapaph K, Rattanakaemakorn P, et al. Six-year retrospective review of drug reaction with eosinophilia and systemic symptoms. Acta Derm Venereol 2012;92:200–5.

29. Mehta U, Maartens G. Is it safe to switch between efavirenz and nevirapine in the event of toxicity? Lancet Infect Dis 2007;7:733–8.

30. Raviglione MC, Narain JP, Kochi A. HIV-associated tuberculosis in developing countries: clinical features, diagnosis, and treatment. Bull World Health Organ 1992;70:515–26.

31. Bigby M. Rates of cutaneous reactions to drugs. Arch Dermatol 2001;137:765–70.

32. Martinez E, Collazos J, Mayo J. Hypersensitivity reactions to rifampin. Pathogenetic mechanisms, clinical manifestations, management strategies, and review of the anaphylactic-like reactions. Medicine (Baltimore) 1999;78:361–9.

33. Roujeau JC. Clinical heterogeneity of drug hypersensitivity. Toxicology 2005;209:123–9.

34. Nunn P, Kibuga D, Gathua S, et al. Cutaneous hypersensitivity reactions due to thiacetazone in HIV-1 seropositive patients treated for tuberculosis. Lancet 1991;337:627–30.

35. Nunn P, Gicheha C, Hayes R, et al. Cross-sectional survey of HIV infection among patients with tuberculosis in Nairobi, Kenya. Tuber Lung Dis 1992;73:45–51.

36. Kardaun SH, Sekula P, Valeyrie-Allanore L, et al. Drug Reaction with Eosinophilia and Systemic Symptoms (DRESS): an original multisystem adverse drug reaction. Results from the prospective RegiSCAR study. Br J Dermatol 2013;169(5):1071–80.

37. Walsh S, Diaz-Cano S, Higgins E, et al. Drug reaction with eosinophilia and systemic symptoms: is cutaneous phenotype a prognostic marker for outcome? A review of clinicopathological features of 27 cases. Br J Dermatol 2013;168:391–401.

38. Akhyani M, Ghodsi ZS, Toosi S, et al. Erythroderma: a clinical study of 97 cases. BMC Dermatol 2005;5:5.

39. Egbers RG, Do TT, Su L, et al. Rapid clinical change in lesions of atypical cutaneous lymphoproliferative disorder in an HIV patient: a case report and review of the literature. Dermatol Online J 2011;17:4.

40. Morar N, Willis-Owen SA, Maurer T, et al. HIV-associated psoriasis: pathogenesis, clinical features, and management. Lancet Infect Dis 2010;10:470–8.

41. Munyao TM, Abinya NA, Ndele JK, et al. Exfoliative erythroderma at Kenyatta National Hospital, Nairobi. East Afr Med J 2007;84:566–70.

42. Zhang P, Chiriboga L, Jacobson M, et al. Mycosis fungoideslike T-cell cutaneous lymphoid infiltrates in patients with HIV infection. Am J Dermatopathol 1995;17:29–35.

43. Husain Z, Reddy BY, Schwartz RA. DRESS syndrome: part II. Management and therapeutics. J Am Acad Dermatol 2013;68:709.e1–9 [quiz: 718–20].

44. Chen YC, Chiu HC, Chu CY. Drug reaction with eosinophilia and systemic symptoms: a retrospective study of 60 cases. Arch Dermatol 2010;146:1373–9.

45. Chiou CC, Yang LC, Hung SI, et al. Clinicopathological features and prognosis of drug rash with eosinophilia and systemic symptoms: a study of 30 cases in Taiwan. J Eur Acad Dermatol Venereol 2008;22:1044–9.

46. Chen YC, Chang CY, Cho YT, et al. Long-term sequelae of drug reaction with eosinophilia and systemic symptoms: a retrospective cohort study from Taiwan. J Am Acad Dermatol 2013;68:459–65.

47. Mittmann N, Knowles SR, Koo M, et al. Incidence of toxic epidermal necrolysis and Stevens-Johnson Syndrome in an HIV cohort: an observational, retrospective case series study. Am J Clin Dermatol 2012;13:49–54.

48. de Prost N, Ingen-Housz-Oro S, Duong T, et al. Bacteremia in Stevens-Johnson syndrome and toxic epidermal necrolysis: epidemiology, risk factors, and predictive value of skin cultures. Medicine (Baltimore) 2010;89:28–36.

49. Ghislain PD, Roujeau JC. Treatment of severe drug reactions: Stevens-Johnson syndrome, toxic epidermal necrolysis and hypersensitivity syndrome. Dermatol Online J 2002;8:5.

50. Lee HY, Dunant A, Sekula P, et al. The role of prior corticosteroid use on the clinical course of Stevens-Johnson syndrome and toxic epidermal necrolysis: a case-control analysis of patients selected from the multinational EuroSCAR and RegiSCAR studies. Br J Dermatol 2012;167:555–62.

51. Mockenhaupt M. The current understanding of Stevens-Johnson syndrome and toxic epidermal necrolysis. Expert Rev Clin Immunol 2011;7:803–13 [quiz: 814–5].

52. Mockenhaupt M, Roujeau JC. Use of high dose intravenous immunoglobulins in dermatology. J Dtsch Dermatol Ges 2010;8:386–7 [author reply: 387–9].

53. De Rojas MV, Dart JK, Saw VP. The natural history of Stevens Johnson syndrome: patterns of chronic ocular disease and the role of systemic immunosuppressive therapy. Br J Ophthalmol 2007;91:1048–53.

54. Misra SP, Dwivedi M, Misra V. Esophageal stricture as a late sequel of Stevens-Johnson syndrome in adults: incidental detection because of foreign body impaction. Gastrointest Endosc 2004;59:437–40.

55. Meneux E, Paniel BJ, Pouget F, et al. Vulvovaginal sequelae in toxic epidermal necrolysis. J Reprod Med 1997;42:153–6.

56. Murphy MI, Brant WE. Hematocolpos caused by genital bullous lesions in a patient with Stevens-Johnson syndrome. J Clin Ultrasound 1998;26:52–4.

57. Samanci N, Balci N, Alpsoy E. Heterotopic ossification related to toxic epidermal necrolysis in a patient with Behcet's disease. J Dermatol 2005;32:469–73.

58. Lehloenya RJ, Todd G, Mogotlane L, et al. Lichenoid drug reaction to antituberculosis drugs treated through with topical steroids and phototherapy. J Antimicrob Chemother 2012;67:2535–7.

59. Valeyrie-Allanore L, Sassolas B, Roujeau JC. Drug-induced skin, nail and hair disorders. Drug Saf 2007;30:1011–30.

60. Chantachaeng W, Chularojanamontri L, Kulthanan K, et al. Cutaneous adverse reactions to sulfonamide antibiotics. Asian Pac J Allergy Immunol 2011;29:284–9.

61. Smith KJ, Yeager J, Skelton H. Fixed drug eruptions to human immunodeficiency virus-1 protease inhibitor. Cutis 2000;66:29–32.

62. Isaacs T, Ngwanya MR, Dlamini S, et al. Annular erythema and photosensitivity as manifestations of efavirenz-induced cutaneous reactions: a review of five consecutive cases. J Antimicrob Chemother 2013;68(12):2871–4.

63. Lehloenya RJ, Isaacs T, Dlamini S, et al. Cutaneous adverse drug reactions caused by FDCAs - we need to characterise and manage them urgently. S Afr Med J 2013;103(11):815.

64. Studer M, Waton J, Bursztejn AC, et al. Does hypersensitivity to multiple drugs really exist? Ann Dermatol Venereol 2012;139:375–80 [in French].

65. Lehloenya RJ, Wallace J, Todd G, et al. Multiple drug hypersensitivity reactions to anti-tuberculosis drugs: five cases in HIV-infected patients. Int J Tuberc Lung Dis 2012;16:1260–4.

66. Shiohara T, Kurata M, Mizukawa Y, et al. Recognition of immune reconstitution syndrome necessary for better management of patients with severe drug eruptions and those under immunosuppressive therapy. Allergol Int 2010;59:333–43.

67. Lehloenya R, Meintjes G. Dermatologic manifestations of the immune reconstitution inflammatory syndrome. Dermatol Clin 2006;24:549–70, vii.

68. Shebe K, Ngwanya M, Gantsho N, et al. Severe recurrence of drug rash with eosinophilia and systemic symptoms secondary to rifampicin patch testing in a human immunodeficiecy virus-infected man. Contact Dermatitis, in press.

69. Adam J, Pichler WJ, Yerly D. Delayed drug hypersensitivity: models of T-cell stimulation. Br J Clin Pharmacol 2011;71:701–7.

70. Bera E, Mia R. Safety of Nevirapine in HIV- infected pregnant women initiating antiretroviral therapy at higher CD4 counts: a systematic review and meta- analysis. S Afr Med J 2012;102(11):1–15.

71. Stewart A, Boulle A, de Waal A, et al. Antiretroviral-associated severe cutaneous adverse drug reactions. Unpublished paper presented the Department of Medicine Research Day, University of Cape Town. Cape Town, South Africa, October 3, 2013.

72. Mayston R, Kinyanda E, Chishinga N, et al. Mental disorder and the outcome of HIV/AIDS in low-income and middle-income countries: a systematic review. AIDS 2012;26(suppl 2):S117–35.

73. Zitha E, Chiliza B, Muloiwa R, et al. Incidence of anxiety and depression in a predominantly HIV-infected population with severe adverse skin reactions. Unpublished paper presented the 66th Congress of the Dermatological Society of South Africa. Cape Town, South Africa, August 31, 2013.

Infective Dermatitis Associated with HTLV-1 Mimics Common Eczemas in Children and May Be a Prelude to Severe Systemic Diseases

Carol Hlela, PhD, MD[a],*, Achiléa Bittencourt, MD[b]

KEYWORDS

- Infective dermatitis • Atopic dermatitis • Seborrhoeic dermatitis • HTLV-1 infection
- Adult T cell leukemia/lymphoma (ATLL)

KEY POINTS

- The variable clinical presentation of IDH, in particular its chronicity, the morphology and distribution of the lesions, and its clinical resemblance to other cutaneous inflammatory conditions, make it hard to distinguish from other common dermatoses.
- It is important to know which factors lead only some infected children to develop IDH and how to prevent the progression of IDH to HAM/TSP and adult T-cell leukemia/lymphoma (ATLL), which in some areas occurs very early.
- Considering that IDH and ATLL occur through vertical transmission of HTLV-1, it is important to prevent this route of transmission.

INTRODUCTION

Human T-cell lymphotropic virus type 1 (HTLV-1), the first isolated human pathogenic retrovirus, was discovered independently in Japan and the United States. In Japan in 1977, Uchiyama and colleagues[1] described a human malignant disease termed adult T-cell leukemia/lymphoma (ATLL). Three years later, in 1980 in the United States, the identification of the first human retrovirus was reported, human T-cell leukemia virus type-1 (HTLV-1) in a patient with cutaneous T-cell lymphoma.[2] Concurrently, the virus was also isolated by Yoshida and colleagues[3] and was termed adult T-cell leukemia virus (ATLV). Soon, HTLV and ATLV were shown to be identical at the sequence[3] level and have since been named HTLV type 1.[4]

Subsequent molecular studies confirmed HTLV-1 as the etiological agent for ATLL[5] and that the virus encodes a 40-kDa cell-transforming oncoprotein named Tax (Transactivator X).[4] Later, another HTLV was isolated, human T-cell lymphotropic virus type-2 (HTLV-2).[6] Both viruses are similar in 66% of their genome sequences and because of this, there are serologic cross-reactions between them. HTLV-2 has not been consistently linked with any given pathology; however, there are few publications that have related it to neurologic diseases.[7]

THE ORIGINS OF HTLV-1

HTLV-1 infection in humans may have had more than one origin. The major origin is thought to be

No conflict of interest.

[a] Division of Dermatology, Red Cross War Memorial Children's Hospital, University of Cape Town, Klipfontein Road, Rondebosch, Cape Town, Western Cape 7700, South Africa; [b] Laboratory Service, Complexo Hospitalar Universita'rio Prof Edgars Santos, University of Bahia, Rua Augusto Viana, s/n-Canela-40110-160 Salvador, Bahia, Brazil

* Corresponding author.

E-mail address: carol.hlela@uct.ac.za

derm.theclinics.com

in equatorial Africa in primates and chimpanzees carrying a virus closely related to HTLV-1. It is likely that this represents the source of virus in descendants of people who came to the Americas (the Caribbean Islands, United States, and South America) from Africa. There is also evidence that the virus could have come to Japan with European voyagers and travelers who took with them people and primates from Africa. As discussed further below, HTLV-1 varies little when contrasted with HIV. Nonetheless, there are variants that exist within populations. Variants from humans are closely related to variants of African chimpanzees.

GEOGRAPHIC SUBTYPES

Six different genetic subtypes of HTLV-1 have been proposed based on phylogenetic analyses: a, or Cosmopolitan, which is distributed worldwide; b, from Central Africa; c, a highly divergent Melanesian strain from Papua Guinea and Australia; d, isolated from Central African Republic pygmies, and from 2 patients in Cameroon and Gabon; e, isolated in a single sample from an Efe pygmy in the Democratic Republic of Congo; and subtype f, detected in an individual from Gabon. The most widespread and best studied subtype, Cosmopolitan, is further divided into 5 subgroups based on geographic distribution: (A) Transcontinental, (B) Japanese, (C) West African/Caribbean, (D) North African, and (E) Black Peruvian. The most widespread (with a worldwide distribution) and best studied is the Cosmopolitan subtype A (HTLV-1 a), which is also the strain prevalent in South Africa.[8] There is no association between the subtypes and clinical manifestations.

HTLV-1 TRANSMISSION

Modes of transmission are shared between the HTLVs and HIVs. Transmission typically occurs horizontally through blood contact, including the transfusion of infected cellular products or the sharing of needles and syringes,[9] but also sexually through the transfer of contaminated body fluids. Vertical transmission occurs primarily during breastfeeding and only rarely in utero. The efficiency of the mother-to-child transmission route is estimated to be 20% and has been correlated with individual variables, such as HTLV-1 proviral load, the concordance of HLA class I type between mother and child, and the duration of breastfeeding.[10] Mother-to-child transmission during the intrauterine period or peripartum has been reported to occur in fewer than 5% of cases.[11]

Similar to other sexually transmitted infections, sexual transmission of HTLV-1 is associated with unprotected sex,[12] multiple sexual partners, lifetime contact with an HTLV-1–infected partner, the presence of genital sores or ulcers, and paying or receiving money for sex. The route of infection has been shown to be related to the development of specific diseases associated with HTLV-1. For example, ATLL has been associated with breastfeeding[11] and HTLV-1–associated myelopathy/tropical spastic paraparesis (HAM/TSP) with blood transfusion[13] and breastfeeding.[14] Rare cases of posttransfusion ATLL have been described.[15] The risk of HTLV-1 transmission by transfusion varies with the prevalence of the virus in the general population, as well as in blood donors. The time interval before seroconversion is also another important variable that interferes with the calculation of the residual risk of transmission. In the case of transfusion-transmitted HTLV-1, the window period usually varies between 41 and 65 days but may be longer.[16]

CLINICAL CHARACTERISTICS OF HTLV-1 INFECTION

The most widely known clinical entities associated with HTLV-1 are ATLL, HAM/TSP,[17,18] HTLV-1–associated uveitis (HAU),[19] and infective dermatitis associated with HTLV-1 (IDH).[20] Most infected individuals remain asymptomatic throughout life, aptly named asymptomatic carriers (ACs). Generally, it is considered that only 2% to 5%[21] of infected individuals develop an HTLV-1–related clinical disorder.[22,23] Notwithstanding, there is increasing evidence that HTLV-1 infection is responsible either directly or indirectly, for a variety of other diseases, including arthropathy, periodontal disease, sicca syndrome, Sjögren's syndrome, polymyositis, lymphocytic alveolitis, and a large number of neurologic deficits. It is particularly striking that these findings occur in a large group of individuals traditionally considered to be asymptomatic HTLV-1 carriers, indicating that morbidity associated with HTLV-1 is much higher than has been generally considered.[24,25] HTLV-1 is an indolent virus with a long latency period between infection and development of disease.[26,27] Individuals infected by HTLV-1 are more susceptible to other infections, such as tuberculosis and other bacterial infections, viral infections, and superficial mycoses. They also present frequently with parasitoses, such as scabies, including crusted scabies and strongyloidiasis, with a high risk of disseminated strongyloidiasis.[25,28]

DIAGNOSIS OF HTLV-1 INFECTION

The most commonly used method for the diagnosis of HTLV-1 infection is serology and the most used serologic screening test is the enzyme-linked immunosorbent assay (ELISA). Samples that repeatedly test positive in the ELISA must be retested in an immunoblot assay for serologic confirmation so as to distinguish between HTLV-1 and HTLV-2.[26] The preferentially used immunoblot assay is the highly sensitive Western blot 2.4. Cases that do not meet the criteria for HTLV-1 or HTLV-2 positivity are considered indeterminate. In these cases, molecular testing should be carried out, polymerase chain reaction (PCR) being the most commonly used method capable of clarifying indeterminate serologic status. This method may even detect infection in individuals who were defined as seronegative but who had a clinical status suggestive of HTLV-1–associated disease. PCR is also used to detect DNA in tumor tissues and in other biologic specimens.

IMMUNE CONTROL OF HTLV-1 INFECTION

HTLV-1's lifelong persistence in CD4$^+$ lymphocytes determines a prolonged interaction between the virus and the immune system, which may ultimately result in a broad spectrum of associated diseases. The immunopathogenic mechanism behind this may be related to the direct action of the virus on the immune system or a consequence of the response of the immune system to the virus. Instead of immunosuppression, HTLV-1 infection causes dysregulation of the immune system with spontaneous lymphoproliferation and increased T-cell activation. Unstimulated cells from asymptomatic HTLV-1 carriers have been shown to secrete high levels of Th1 and Th2 cytokines, such as tumor necrosis factor alfa (TNF-α), interferon-γ (IFN-γ), and interleukin (IL)-5 and IL-10, compared with cells from seronegative individuals.[29] Moreover, it has been found that CD4$^+$ lymphocytes represent the principal source of IFN-gamma and that high levels of IL-10 are able to down-regulate the exacerbated Th1-type immune response that occurs in these carriers.[29]

Mechanisms underlying the persistence and pathogenesis of HTLV-1 remain largely unknown; however, factors thought to influence the outcome of HTLV-1 infection include the host's immune response,[30] gene expression in host lymphocytes,[31] the genomic integration site,[32] and the sequence of the provirus.[33]

The role of the innate immune response in persistent HTLV-1 infection is unclear. It seems that persistence of the virus in the skin or blood may be partly the result of the inadequate immune response.[34] The question is, therefore, how much does the failed innate immune response influence the role and the extent to which the adaptive immune response responds to the presence of the virus.

There has been a longstanding debate on the question of whether HTLV-1 is latent or persistently expressed in vivo.[35] Persistent expression, instead of latency, is slowly gaining acceptance.[36] Speculation has it that HTLV-1 persists through an equilibrium "set point" of proviral HTLV-1, set by a balance between spontaneous proviral expression and cytotoxic T lymphocyte (CTL)-mediated immune surveillance.[37] The variation in the set point among hosts referred to in the previous sections may be explained by 2 possible factors: the rate of proliferation of T cells in response to HTLV-1 expression driven mainly by Tax protein, and the rate at which CTLs kill HTLV-1–expressing cells. It has been observed that individual clones of infected cells can persist in patients for several years,[38] indicating that the proviral load (PVL) is maintained in vivo mainly by infected cells undergoing mitosis during the chronic phase of infection. This leads to the hypothesis that infectious transmission of HTLV-1 is important early in infection across the virological synapse,[31,39] whereas mitotic replication is responsible for maintaining PVL once a persistent infection has been established and has reached equilibrium with the immune response.[40] In up to 5% of infected individuals, persistent clonal proliferation culminates in malignant transformation in ATLL.[41,42] The leukemic clones generally carry only one (complete or defective) provirus per cell.[33,43] Evidence has shown that within a given HTLV-1–infected individual, 2 features differentiate the clones of infected cells: the antigenic specificity of the T-cell clones (eg, T-cell receptors), and epigenetic modifications or the proviral insertion site in the host genome.[40] Activation of the infected T cell by either antigen or cytokines (such as IL-2 or IL-15) might result in expression of the integrated provirus.[40] Epigenetic changes in the infected cell affect the rate of proviral infection. The character of the genomic site appears to influence PVL expression,[44] in turn resulting in simultaneously strong positive and negative selection of the T cell. The net effect determines the T cell's survival in the host, and so its contribution to retroviral persistence.

IDH

IDH has been reported in the Caribbean area,[20] Latin America,[44] and in a few countries in Africa, including Senegal and South Africa.[45] The first description of this disease was by Sweet in 1966.[20,46] This investigator recognized 17 patients from Jamaica that had a peculiar type of eczema generally starting at the age of 2 years, seldom before 18 months. The lesions were scaly, exudative, and crusted and distributed on nostrils, ears, face, scalp, and neck. Sweet[46] also observed a generalized and fine papular eruption and the relapsing character of the lesions after withdrawal of antibiotics. In the following year, Walshe[47] documented a high incidence of *Staphylococcus* and/or beta hemolytic *Streptococcus* (BHS) infection in the nose and skin lesions of 25 cases of infective dermatitis.[5,47] It was postulated that these children might be immunosuppressed. In 1990, for the first time infective dermatitis was linked to HTLV-1 infection.[48] This relationship was later confirmed in a study in which 50 patients with IDH were compared with 35 patients with atopic dermatitis (AD).[20] Only 5 of 35 patients with AD were seropositive for HTLV-1. In both groups, microbiologic studies showed frequent colonization with *Staphylococcus aureus* and/or BHS. On comparing the blood count findings between the 2 groups, patients with infective dermatitis were anemic, had a higher white blood cell count and had a more elevated erythrocyte sedimentation rate than patients with AD. They also had a significantly higher incidence of abnormal serum proteins and dermatopathic lymphadenopathy.[20] In this study, the disease was named as IDH and the major and minor criteria for the diagnosis were proposed.[20] Although highly accepted to this day, La Grenade and colleagues'[19] criteria was modified after a follow-up study of 42 infanto-juvenile IDH patients (**Box 1**).[44] The following markers expand from La Grenade and colleagues' original criteria.

1. No reference was made in La Grenade and colleagues' criteria to the frequency of the affected areas and, as such, it is important to consider that the scalp is always involved. In Bahia, Brazil, besides the scalp, the retroauricular areas are also involved in 100% of the cases and in all patients at least 3 areas are affected.
2. Crusting of the nostrils was a common finding; however, this feature was absent in some patients, and it is an inconstant feature.
3. Rhinorrhea is a common symptom in children caused by several other diseases.
4. The relapsing nature of this disease with a prompt response to appropriate therapy and an equally rapid relapse if the drugs are withdrawn, was present in all the patients and should be considered as an indispensable criterion for diagnosis.

Box 1
Major criteria for the diagnosis of infective dermatitis associated with HTLV-1

1. Presence of erythematous-scaly, exudative, and crusted lesions of the scalp, retroauricular areas, neck, axillae, groin, paranasal and perioral skin, ears, thorax, abdomen, and other sites
2. Crusting of nostrils
3. Chronic relapsing dermatitis with prompt response to appropriate therapy but prompt recurrence on discontinuation of treatment
4. Diagnosis of HTLV-1 infection (by serologic or molecular biologic testing)

Of the 4 major criteria, 3 are required for diagnosis, with mandatory inclusion of numbers 1, 3, and 4. To fulfill criteria 1, involvement of ≥3 of the sites is required, including involvement of the scalp and retroauricular areas.
Abbreviation: HTLV-1, human T-cell lymphotropic virus type-1.
From De Oliveira MD, Fatal PL, Primo JR, et al. Infective dermatitis associated with human T-cell lymphotropic virus type 1: evaluation of 42 cases observed in Bahia, Brazil. Clin Infect Dis 2012;54(12):1718; with permission.

---

5. The disease may begin later in childhood, and even in adulthood.
6. In some patients serologically negative for HTLV-1, PCR performed in peripheral blood mononuclear cells may be positive, and it is prudent to test when patients with the classic characteristics of IDH present negative serology.[44]

IDH has been correlated with vertical transmission and long-term breastfeeding.[44,48] Furthermore, IDH may represent an early clinical marker for HTLV-1 infection and an indicator of increased risk for developing other, even more devastating HTLV-1–associated diseases.

CLINICAL FINDINGS

The disease generally appears at 18 months but may occur earlier. In one study, in 37% of the patients the disease appeared at 12 months or earlier.[44] The frequency of IDH is greater among female patients.[20,44] IDH is a chronic and recurrent eczema occurring during childhood and infrequently in adolescence or adulthood. It is distinctive, often beginning with a rhinitis identified by the mother as a "cold." This is followed by an oozing, weeping eruption on many body areas.[49] The lesions are erythematous, scaly, frequently covered by yellow and fetid crusts always involving the scalp (**Fig. 1**), retroauricular

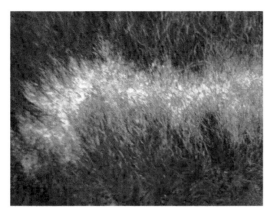

Fig. 1. Diffuse erythematous-scaly lesion on the scalp covered by yellow crusts. (*Courtesy of* Dr Maria de Fátima Paim, MD, Federal University of Bahia, Brazil.)

regions (**Fig. 2**), and many other areas (**Figs. 3** and **4, Table 1**), sometimes associated with other types of skin or mucosal lesions (**Table 2**). In one study, the lesions were disseminated in 83% of the patients.[44,46] As previously referred, affected individuals have to fulfill the major criteria for a diagnosis to be made (see **Box 1**). S aureus and/or BHS are generally cultured from the anterior nares or skin lesions. Patients who had no treatment for a period of more than 6 months and who presented no skin lesions are considered to be in remission.[44] The mean age of complete remission of IDH is 15 years, varying from 10 to 20 years.[44] However, IDH has been reported to persist until 23 years of age.[44] It is important to emphasize that IDH may begin in adulthood with the same clinical and immunohistochemical characteristics of IDH at early onset. However, there are only 9 reported cases, all in female patients and 4 associated with HAM/TSP.[47,50] Comorbidities associated with IDH include scabies,

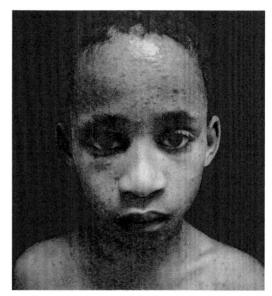

Fig. 3. Erythematous-scaly lesion with small crusts on the scalp and the external ear with small papules on the face. (*Courtesy of* Dr Maria de Fátima Paim, MD, Federal University of Bahia, Brazil.)

corneal opacities, acquired icthiosis, chronic bronchiectasis, glomerulonephritis, and lymphocytic interstitial pneumonitis.[44,45,49,51]

DIFFERENTIAL DIAGNOSIS

The most important differential diagnosis of IDH is with AD (**Table 3**).[19,44,52] A positive serology for HTLV-1, although helpful, is not the only criterion for diagnosis.[19] Both diseases are susceptible to infection of the lesions by S aureus; however, infection is more marked in IDH. A childhood onset is also shared by the 2 conditions but a significant

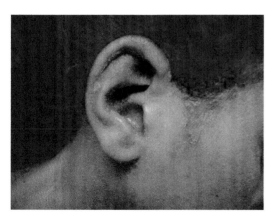

Fig. 2. Erythematous-scaly lesion on the scalp, the retroauricular area, and the posterior aspect of the neck. (*Courtesy of* Dr Maria de Fátima Paim, MD, Federal University of Bahia, Brazil.)

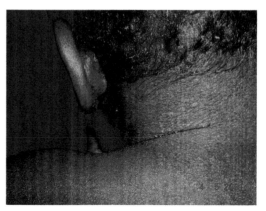

Fig. 4. Crusted lesion on the scalp. Erythematous-scaly lesions on the eyebrows, ears, paranasal skin, perioral region, and neck. Small papules on the forehead. (*Courtesy of* Dr Maria de Fátima Paim, MD, Federal University of Bahia, Brazil.)

Table 1
Distribution of lesions in 42 patients with infective dermatitis associated with human T-cell lymphotropic virus type-1 from Bahia, Brazil

Lesion Location	n (%)
Scalp	42 (100)
Retroauricular regions	42 (100)
Neck	37 (88.1)
Axillae	35 (83.3)
Groin	33 (78.6)
Paranasal skin	30 (71.4)
Ears	30 (71.4)
Thorax	27 (64.3)
Abdomen	26 (61.9)
Antecubital and popliteal fossae	24 (57.1)
Eyelids	24 (57.1)
Forehead	23 (54.8)
Perioral region	21 (50.0)
Umbilicus	17 (40.5)
Limbs	15 (35.7)
External genitalia	14 (33.3)
Buttocks	7 (16.7)

From De Oliveira MD, Fatal PL, Primo JR, et al. Infective dermatitis associated with human T-cell lymphotropic virus type 1: evaluation of 42 cases observed in Bahia, Brazil. Clin Infect Dis 2012;54(12):1715; with permission.

difference between these conditions is the absence of family history of atopy in IDH, a feature that characterizes AD. Patients with both conditions complain of pruritus, even though the

Table 2
Frequency of lesions in infective dermatitis associated with human T-cell lymphotropic virus in 42 patients from Bahia, Brazil

Type of Condition	n (%)
Erythematous-scaly-crusty lesions	42 (100)
Retroauricular fissures	32 (76.2)
Slightly erythematous-scaly papules	32 (76.2)
Crusting of nostrils	27 (64.3)
Fine papular rash	25 (59.5)
Blepharoconjunctivitis	24 (57.1)
Follicular papules	19 (45.2)

From De Oliveira MD, Fatal PL, Primo JR, et al. Infective dermatitis associated with human T-cell lymphotropic virus type 1: evaluation of 42 cases observed in Bahia, Brazil. Clin Infect Dis 2012;54(12):1717; with permission.

intensity is much less in IDH.[44,46] Different from AD, patients with IDH always present severe lesions in the scalp and retroauricular regions, frequently with retroauricular fissures. On the other hand, the frequent findings of lesions in the antecubital and popliteal fossae may sometimes make it difficult the differentiate IDH from AD.[44,46,48,51] The main differential diagnosis is clinical and is accessible to all dermatologists.

Differential diagnosis with seborrhoeic dermatitis (SD) is imperative only when the IDH begins in puberty, which occurs infrequently. SD is more common during or after puberty, the time during which IDH improves or disappears. Although there are some similarities, IDH has distinct clinical features that allow for it to be differentiated from SD (**Table 4**).[19,44,53] In IDH, the cutaneous lesions tend to be more prominent, more exudative, and markedly infected. IDH promptly responds to appropriate therapy, but relapses on discontinuation of antibiotics or sulfonamides.[5,44] On the other hand, crusting of the anterior nares and a disseminated papular rash are observed only in IDH. In addition, *Pityrosporum* yeasts, known to occur frequently in seborrheic dermatitis, are not observed in the lesions of IDH.[44]

PATHOLOGIC AND IMMUNOHISTOCHEMICAL FINDINGS

The pathologic aspects of IDH are similar to other types of eczema, such as AD and SD, predominantly being those of a spongiotic dermatitis of variable degrees of intensity or of a simple chronic dermatitis, depending on the duration of the biopsied lesion. Thus, pathology does not help in the differential diagnosis among IDH, AD, or SD. Infrequently, histology may mimic psoriasis or mycosis fungoides.[54] Biopsies for immunohistochemical findings are important. In contrast to what is observed in AD and SD, in which the T lymphocytes are predominantly of the helper cell phenotype, in IDH the infiltrate is only or predominantly CD8 positive.[54] Nevertheless, the CD8-positive lymphocytes are perforin negative and rarely granzyme-B[+], suggesting that they are not activated cytotoxic T lymphocytes.[54]

DISEASE EVOLUTION

Epidemiologic data suggest that IDH is not only a marker of childhood HTLV-1 infection but also a possible harbinger of more serious HTLV-1–associated disorders.[55] Reports indicate that IDH increases an individual's risk for ATLL and HAM/TSP.[56,57]

Table 3
Different clinical characteristics of infective dermatitis associated with HTLV-1 and atopic dermatitis up to 18 months

Clinical Characteristic	IDH	AD
Age at onset	From 18–24 mo onward	From 18–24 mo onward
Atopy	Absent	Present
Pruritus	Slight to moderate	Severe
Skin lesions	Erythematous-scaly lesions with yellow crusts, papules, retroauricular fissures, and generalized fine papular rash	Erythematous and edematous papules and plaques, sometimes with vesiculation, generally replaced by lichenification
Distribution	Scalp, retroauricular areas, external ear, eyelids margins, perinasal skin, neck, axillae, and groin	Elbow and knee flexures, sides of the neck, wrists, ankles, and hands
Crusting on anterior nares	Present	Absent
Blepharoconjunctivitis	Present	Absent

Abbreviations: AD, atopic dermatitis; HTLV-1, human T-cell lymphotropic virus type-1; IDH, infective dermatitis associated with HTLV-1.
Data from Refs.[19,44,52]

ATLL is an aggressive lymphoproliferative malignancy of peripheral T cells, with short survival in its acute form. It is classified into 5 clinical forms: acute, chronic, lymphoma, smoldering (leukemic and non-leukemic), and primary cutaneous tumoral.[20,58] Its occurrence is associated with vertical transmission of HTLV-1 through breastfeeding.[11] There are rare reports about progression of IDH to ATLL in puberty.[59–61] It has been observed that 37.5% of cases of ATLL with cutaneous manifestations have had a history of severe childhood eczema involving the scalp that was suggestive of IDH.[62]

The mechanisms that lead to this development have not yet been elucidated. It is probable that both genetic factors of the host and external factors are involved.

Table 4
Different clinical characteristics of infective dermatitis associated with HTLV-1 and seborrheic dermatitis

Clinical Characteristic	IDH	SD
Age at onset	From 18 mo onward	Puberty and adulthood
Pruritus	Slight to moderate	Severe
Skin lesions	Erythematous-scaly lesions with yellow crusts, papules, retroauricular fissures, and generalized fine papular rash	Erythematous greasy scaly lesions
Distribution	Scalp, retroauricular areas, external ear, eyelids margins, perinasal skin, neck, axillae, thorax, abdomen, and groin	Scalp; retroauricular areas; external ear; glabella; eyebrows; nasolabial folds; neck; presternal, interscapular, and submammary regions; axillae; groin; and umbilicus
Retroauricular fissures	Present	Present
Crusting on anterior nares	Present	Absent
Blepharoconjunctivitis	Present	Present

Abbreviations: HTLV-1, human T-cell lymphotropic virus type-1; IDH, infective dermatitis associated with HTLV-1; SD, seborrhoeic dermatitis.
Data from Refs.[19,44,53]

Gabet and colleagues[63] studied the HTLV-1 replication over 2 years in a patient with IDH associated with strongyloidiasis. They believe that this parasitosis may predispose HTLV-1 carriers to develop ATLL.[49] They observed elevated PVL together with persistent oligoclonal expansion of the infected lymphocytes. The replication pattern was very different from that observed in asymptomatic carriers, being more similar to the pattern found in ATLL.[64,65]

HAM/TSP is a myelopathy characterized by slowly progressive spastic paraparesis that may cause mild sensory involvement and bladder disturbances. Even though HAM/TSP has been characterized as an adult-onset disease, several cases with early-life onset have been described, most of them associated with IDH.[44,57] Among 36 cases of IDH with continued follow-up, 17 progressed to HAM/TSP in childhood or adolescence.[44]

Additionally, early deaths have also been documented in 5 patients with IDH: 2 in Jamaica at 14 and 19 years of age with ATLL-like syndromes and 3 in Brazil.[44,49] Two of the Brazilian patients had IDH and HAM/TSP and died at 13 and 22 years of age with rheumatic cardiopathy and kidney failure, respectively. The third patient who had abandoned follow-up and was living on the streets, died at 22 years of age of dehydration caused by diarrhea of unknown etiology.[44]

There is a great familial clustering among cases of IDH and of juvenile HAM/TSP.[44,46,51,57] Recently, clustering of IDH and/or HAM/TSP was shown in 15 families observed among 28 families with IDH, of which 93% of the cases occurred in 2 generations. With the exception of 2 mothers of children with IDH, all the mothers with HAM/TSP had at least one child with HAM/TSP.[66]

PATHOGENESIS

HTLV-1 PVL is a major determinant of disease development in infected individuals and is considered to remain stable over time.[52,67] The rate of HTLV-1 proviral expression has been shown to correlate with the outcome of infection. PVL is higher in adulthood HAM/TSP and ATLL in relation to asymptomatic carriers. It has also been observed that the HTLV-1 PVL is significantly higher in patients with IDH than in asymptomatic carriers and is similar to that found in patients with HAM/TSP.[53,68]

According to Gillet and colleagues,[69] the significantly higher PVL in IDH, also observed in carriers with strongiloidiasis, was due to an increase in the mean clone abundance, and not due to an increase in the number of infected clones.

Patients with IDH produce larger quantities of TNF-α and IFN-gamma than HTLV-1 carriers and are able to modulate IFN-gamma production when anti–IL-15 is added.[70] However, anti–IL-2 was not able to significantly reduce the immunologic response in these patients.[70] These data indicate that IDH is characterized by an exaggerated, type-1 immune response. Furthermore, no difference was observed between mRNA in IDH and controls, which supports the findings that an immunologic response in IDH differs from AD and that a type-2 immune response is not responsible for the tissue damage observed in IDH.[70] The similarities between the immunologic response in patients with IDH and HAM/TSP and the high PVL observed in IDH provide support that IDH is a risk factor for development of HAM/TSP.[54,70] TNF-α has been associated with pathology of chronic inflammatory and autoimmune diseases and may be, at least in part, responsible for the marked inflammatory aspect of IDH lesions.

Currently, little is known about the mechanism by which IDH is followed by ATLL later in life in some patients. It is possible that the presence of viral antigens and bacterial superantigens may stimulate the lymphocytes, increasing the number of target cells available to be infected by HTLV-1. With this expansion of infected T-cells, activation signals and growth factors are produced for uninfected T-cells and repeated clonal expansion of these cells increases the chance of the additional events required for transformation and leukemogenesis.[55,71] Recently published data reveal that both the proviral integration sites and the oligoclonality index differ between patients with IDH and those with ATLL.[56,69] Atypical T cells, including flower cells, have been found in peripheral blood smears of 35% (11/31) of patients with IDH (children and adolescents).[72] These cells can be found in adult HTLV-1 carriers considered to be at high risk for developing ATLL. Flower cells are commonly found in the acute-type of ATLL and occasionally in the chronic and smoldering types.[72] Moreover, proviral monoclonal integration was detected in 7 of those 11 patients with IDH with atypical cells in peripheral blood but analysis of T-cell receptor gene rearrangements revealed a polyclonal population of T cells.[73] Furthermore, they cannot be considered as a smoldering form of ATLL because they do not have lymphoma or 5% or more of atypical cells in peripheral blood. These children represent pre-ATLL cases and are probably at a greater risk of developing ATLL. The pre-ATLL condition has been reported in 1.7% of asymptomatic adult carriers and 42% of them progressed to ATLL.[74]

TREATMENT AND PREVENTION OF COMPLICATIONS

Because IDH is always associated with bacterial infection, treatment of IDH is currently aimed at controlling infection by *S aureus* and BHS. A treatment with sulfamethoxazole-trimethoprim (40 mg/kg/d of sulfamethoxazole and 8 mg/kg/d of trimethoprim) for 15 days and thereafter, one-half dose at night until the disease is controlled, has been recommended.[48,51] Erythromycin was used to treat one child who was allergic to sulfonamides and had an excellent response.[51] Good results are being obtained in the Dermatologic Clinics of the Federal University of Bahia using cephalexin (50 mg/kg/d) for 10 days before the use of the sulfur drugs Generally, the treatment lasts 3 to 12 months, depending on the response. If a relapse occurs during treatment, a complete dose must be restarted (Bittencourt AL, personal communication, 2013).

A combination of prophylactic immunoglobulin and perhaps antiretroviral therapy need to be investigated for possible use in the control of infection. Some investigators are also exploring the feasibility of an HTLV-1 vaccine.[75,76] It is recommended that these patients be carefully followed with clinical and laboratory examinations.

SUMMARY

As IDH may simulate other childhood cutaneous inflammatory conditions, it is imperative that the pediatricians know its characteristics so as to make a correct diagnosis and provide the correct treatment. These patients must be followed carefully even after disappearance of the cutaneous lesions so as to detect early possible adverse evolutions. Further research is necessary to determine factors that lead to only some infected children developing IDH, mechanisms behind the progression of IDH to HAM/TSP and ATLL, which in some parts of the world occurs very early. Considering that IDH and ATLL occur through vertical transmission of HTLV-1, it is important to prevent this route of transmission.

REFERENCES

1. Uchiyama T, Yodoi J, Sagawa K, et al. Adult T-cell leukemia: clinical and hematologic features of 16 cases. Blood 1977;50:481–92.
2. Poiesz BJ, Ruscetti FW, Gazdar AF, et al. Detection and isolation of type C retrovirus particles from fresh and cultured lymphocytes of a patient with cutaneous T-cell lymphoma. Proc Natl Acad Sci U S A 1980;77:7415–9.
3. Yoshida M, Miyoshi I, Hinuma Y. Isolation and characterization of retrovirus from cell lines of human adult T-cell leukemia and its implication in the disease. Proc Natl Acad Sci U S A 1982;79:2031–5.
4. Gallo RC. History of the discoveries of the first human retroviruses: HTLV-1 and HTLV-2. Oncogene 2005;24:5926–30.
5. Yoshida M, Seiki M. Recent advances in the molecular biology of HTLV-1: trans-activation of viral and cellular genes. Annu Rev Immunol 1987;5:541–59.
6. Yoshida M, Seiki M, Yamaguchi K, et al. Monoclonal integration of human T-cell leukemia provirus in all primary tumors of adult T-cell leukemia suggests causative role of human T-cell leukemia virus in the disease. Proc Natl Acad Sci U S A 1984;81:2534–7.
7. Bittencourt AL, de Oliveira MD. Cutaneous manifestations associated with HTLV-1 infection. Int J Dermatol 2010;49(10):1099–110.
8. Bhigjee AI, Tarin ML, Bill PL, et al. Sequence of the env gene of some KwaZulu-Natal, South African strains of HTLV type I. AIDS Res Hum Retroviruses 1999;15:1229–33.
9. Proietti FA, Carneiro-Proietti AB, Catalan-Soares BC, et al. Global epidemiology of HTLV-I infection and associated diseases. Oncogene 2005;24:6058–68.
10. Biggar RJ, Ng J, Kim N, et al. Human leukocyte antigen concordance and the transmission risk via breast-feeding of human T cell lymphotropic virus type I. J Infect Dis 2006;193:277–82.
11. Fujino T, Nagata Y. HTLV-I transmission from mother to child. J Reprod Immunol 2000;47:197–206.
12. Kaplan JE, Khabbaz RF, Murphy EL, et al. Male-to-female transmission of human T-cell lymphotropic virus types I and II: association with viral load. The Retrovirus Epidemiology Donor Study Group. J Acquir Immune Defic Syndr Hum Retrovirol 1996;12:193–201.
13. Osame M, Janssen R, Kubota H. Nationwide survey of HTLV-1–associated myelopathy in Japan: association with blood transfusion. Ann Neurol 1990;28:50–6.
14. Hanchard B. Outcomes of early life exposure to human T cell lymphotropic virus type 1. Clin Infect Dis 2005;41(4):542–3.
15. Sato H, Okochi K. Transmission of human T-cell leukemia virus (HTLV-I) by blood transfusion: demonstration of proviral DNA in recipients' blood lymphocytes. Int J Cancer 1986;37:395–400.
16. Cruickshank EK. A neuropathic syndrome of uncertain origin; review of 100 cases. West Indian Med J 1956;5:147–58.
17. Gessain A, Barin F, Vernant JC, et al. Antibodies to human T-lymphotropic virus type-I in patients with tropical spastic paraparesis. Lancet 1985;2:407–10.

18. Mochizuki M, Watanabe T, Yamaguchi K, et al. Uveitis associated with human T lymphotropic virus type I: seroepidemiologic, clinical, and virologic studies. J Infect Dis 1992;166:943–4.

19. La Grenade L, Manns A, Fletcher V. Clinical, pathologic, and immunologic features of human T lymphotropic virus type-1 associated infective dermatitis in children. Arch Dermatol 1998;134:439–44.

20. Shimoyama M. Diagnostic criteria and classification of clinical subtypes of adult T-cell leukaemia-lymphoma. A report from the Lymphoma Study Group (1984–87). Br J Haematol 1991;79:428–37.

21. Verdonck K, Gonzalez E, Van Dooren S, et al. Human T-lymphotropic virus 1: recent knowledge about an ancient infection. Lancet Infect Dis 2007;7:266–81.

22. Yakova M, Lézin A, Dantin F, et al. Increased proviral load in HTLV-1-infected patients with rheumatoid arthritis or connective tissue disease. Retrovirology 2005;2:4.

23. Poetker SK, Porto AF, Giozza SP, et al. Clinical manifestations in individuals with recent diagnosis of HTLV type I infection. J Clin Virol 2011;51(1):54–8.

24. Caskey MF, Morgan DJ, Porto AF, et al. Clinical manifestations associated with HTLV type I infection: a cross-sectional study. AIDS Res Hum Retroviruses 2007;23(3):365–71.

25. Manns A, Miley WJ, Wilks RJ, et al. Quantitative proviral DNA and antibody levels in the natural history of HTLV-I infection. J Infect Dis 1999;180:1487–93.

26. Brites C, Weyll M, Pedroso C, et al. Severe and Norwegian scabies are strongly associated with retroviral (HIV-1/HTLV-1) infection in Bahia, Brazil. AIDS 2002;16:1292–3.

27. Bastos MD, Santos SB, Souza A, et al. Influence of HTLV-1 on the clinical, microbiologic and immunologic presentation of tuberculosis. BMC Infect Dis 2012;12:199.

28. Carvalho EM, Bacellar O, Porto AF, et al. Cytokine profile and immunomodulation in asymptomatic human T-lymphotropic virus type 1-infected blood donors. J Acquir Immune Defic Syndr 2001;27:1–6.

29. Komurian F, Pelloquin F, de The G. In vivo genomic variability of human T-cell leukemia virus type I depends more upon geography than upon pathologies. J Virol 1991;65:3770–8.

30. Igakura T, Stinchcombe JC, Goon PK, et al. Spread of HTLV-I between lymphocytes by virus-induced polarization of the cytoskeleton. Science 2003;299:1713–6.

31. Meekings KN, Leipzig J, Bushman FD, et al. HTLV-1 integration into transcriptionally active genomic regions is associated with proviral expression and with HAM/TSP. PLoS Pathog 2008;4:e1000027.

32. Melamed A, Laydon DJ, Gillet NA, et al. Genome-wide determinants of proviral targeting, clonal abundance and expression in natural HTLV-1 infection. PLoS Pathog 2013;9(3):e1003271.

33. Olière S, Douville R, Sze A, et al. Modulation of innate immune responses during human T-cell leukemia virus (HTLV-1) pathogenesis. Cytokine Growth Factor Rev 2011;22(4):197–210.

34. Asquith B, Hanon E, Taylor GP, et al. Is human T-cell lymphotropic virus type I really silent? Philos Trans R Soc Lond B Biol Sci 2000;355:1013–9.

35. Asquith B, Zhang Y, Mosley AJ, et al. In vivo T lymphocyte dynamics in humans and the impact of human T-lymphotropic virus 1 infection. Proc Natl Acad Sci U S A 2007;104:8035–40.

36. Asquith B, Bangham CR. Quantifying HTLV-I dynamics. Immunol Cell Biol 2007;85:280–6.

37. Cavrois M, Leclercq I, Gout O, et al. Persistent oligoclonal expansion of human T-cell leukemia virus type 1-infected circulating cells in patients with tropical spastic paraparesis/HTLV-1 associated myelopathy. Oncogene 1998;17:77–82.

38. Jones KS, Petrow-Sadowski C, Huang YK, et al. Cell-free HTLV-1 infects dendritic cells leading to transmission and transformation of CD4(+) T cells. Nat Med 2008;14:429–36.

39. Bangham CR, Osame M. Cellular immune response to HTLV-1. Oncogene 2005;24:6035–46.

40. Etoh K, Yamaguchi K, Tokudome S, et al. Rapid quantification of HTLV-I provirus load: detection of monoclonal proliferation of HTLV-I-infected cells among blood donors. Int J Cancer 1999;81:859–64.

41. Okayama A, Stuver S, Matsuoka M, et al. Role of HTLV-1 proviral DNA load and clonality in the development of adult T-cell leukemia/lymphoma in asymptomatic carriers. Int J Cancer 2004;110:621–5.

42. Kamihira S, Sugahara K, Tsuruda K, et al. Proviral status of HTLV-1 integrated into the host genomic DNA of adult T-cell leukemia cells. Clin Lab Haematol 2005;27:235–41.

43. Gillet NA, Malani N, Melamed A, et al. The host genomic environment of the provirus determines the abundance of HTLV-1-infected T-cell clones. Blood 2011;117(11):3113–22.

44. De Oliveira Mde F, Fatal PL, Primo JR, et al. Infective dermatitis associated with human T-cell lymphotropic virus type 1: evaluation of 42 cases observed in Bahia, Brazil. Clin Infect Dis 2012;54(12):1714–9.

45. Mahe A, Meertens L, Ly F, et al. Human T-cell leukaemia/lymphoma virus type 1-associated infective dermatitis in Africa: a report of five cases from Senegal. Br J Dermatol 2004;150:958–65.

46. Sweet RD. A pattern of eczema in Jamaica. Br J Dermatol 1966;78:93–100.

47. Walshe MM. Infective dermatitis in Jamaican children. Br J Dermatol 1967;79:229–36.

48. LaGrenade L, Hanchard B, Fletcher V, et al. Infective dermatitis of Jamaican children: a marker for HTLV-I infection. Lancet 1990;336:1345–7.

49. La Grenade L, Schwartz RA, Janniger CK. Childhood dermatitis in the tropics: with special emphasis on infective dermatitis, a marker for infection with human T-cell leukemia virus-I. Cutis 1996;58:115–8.

50. Maragno L, Casseb J, Fukumori LM, et al. Human T-cell lymphotropic virus type 1 infective dermatitis emerging in adulthood. Int J Dermatol 2009;48: 723–30.

51. Oliveira Mde F, Brites C, Ferraz N, et al. Infective dermatitis associated with the human T cell lymphotropic virus type I in Salvador, Bahia, Brazil. Clin Infect Dis 2005;40:e90–6.

52. Friedmann PS, Holden CA. Atopic dermatitis. Chapter 18:29–31. In: Burns T, Breathnach S, Cox N, et al, editors. Rook's textbook of dermatology, vol. 1, 7th edition. Oxford: Blackwell Science Ltd; 2004. p. 29–31.

53. Holden CA, Berth-Jones J. Eczema, lichenification, prurigo and erythroderma. Chapter 17:10–15. In: Burns T, Breathnach S, Cox N, et al, editors. Rook's textbook of dermatology, vol. 1, 7th edition. Oxford: Blackwell Science Ltd; 2004. p. 10–15.

54. Bittencourt AL, Oliveira MF, Brites C. Histological and immunohistological studies of infective dermatitis with HTLV-1. Eur J Dermatol 2005;15: 26–30.

55. Maloney EM, Wiktor SZ, Palmer P, et al. A cohort study of health effects of human T-cell lymphotropic virus type I infection in Jamaican children. Pediatrics 2003;112:e136–42.

56. Araújo AP, Fontenelle LM, Pádua PA, et al. Juvenile human T lymphotropic virus type 1-associated myelopathy. Clin Infect Dis 2002;35(2):201–4.

57. Primo JR, Brites C, Oliveira Mde F, et al. Infective dermatitis and human T cell lymphotropic virus type 1-associated myelopathy/tropical spastic paraparesis in childhood and adolescence. Clin Infect Dis 2005;41:535–41.

58. Bittencourt AL, Barbosa HS, Vieira MG, et al. Adult T-cell leukemia/lymphoma (ATL) in Bahia, Brazil: analysis of prognostic factors in a group of 70 patients. Am J Clin Pathol 2007;128:875–82.

59. Farre L, de Oliveira Mde F, Primo J, et al. Early sequential development of infective dermatitis, human T cell lymphotropic virus type 1-associated myelopathy, and adult T cell leukemia/lymphoma. Clin Infect Dis 2008;46:440–2.

60. Hanchard B, LaGrenade L, Carberry C, et al. Childhood infective dermatitis evolving into adult T-cell leukaemia after 17 years. Lancet 1991; 338:1593–4.

61. Bittencourt A, Brites C, Pereira Filho C, et al. Linfoma/leucemia de células T associado ao HTLV-I (ATL) em criança e adolescente. An Bras Dermatol 2001;76(Suppl 2):88.

62. Bittencourt AL, Barbosa HS, Vieira MD, et al. Adult T-cell leukemia/lymphoma (ATL) presenting in the skin: clinical, histological and immunohistochemical features of 52 cases. Acta Oncol 2009;48: 598–604.

63. Gabet AS, Mortreux F, Talarmin A, et al. High circulating proviral load with oligoclonal expansion of HTLV-1 bearing T cells in HTLV-1 carriers with strongyloidiasis. Oncogene 2000;19: 4954–60.

64. Bittencourt AL, Oliveira Mde F, Ferraz N, et al. Adult-onset infective dermatitis associated with HTLV-I. Clinical and immunopathological aspects of two cases. Eur J Dermatol 2006;16:62–6.

65. Gabet AS, Kazanji M, Couppie P, et al. Adult T-cell leukaemia/lymphoma-like human T-cell leukaemia virus-1 replication in infective dermatitis. Br J Haematol 2003;123:406–12.

66. da Silva JL, Primo JR, de Oliveira MD, et al. Clustering of HTLV-1 associated myelopathy/tropical spastic paraparesis (HAM/TSP) and infective dermatitis associated with HTLV-1 (IDH) in Salvador, Bahia, Brazil. J Clin Virol 2013;1:12–5.

67. Watanabe T. HTLV-1-associated diseases. Int J Hematol 1997;66(3):257–78.

68. Primo J, Siqueira I, Nascimento MC, et al. Patients with infective dermatitis associated with HTLV-1. High HTLV-1 proviral load, a marker for HTLV-1-associated myelopathy/tropical spastic paraparesis, is also detected in patients with infective dermatitis associated with HTLV-1. Braz J Med Biol Res 2009;42(8):761–4.

69. Gillet NA, Cook L, Laydon DJ, et al. Strongyloidiasis and infective dermatitis alter human T lymphotropic virus-1 clonality in vivo. PLoS Pathog 2013; 9(4):e1003263.

70. Nascimento MC, Primo J, Bittencourt A, et al. Infective dermatitis has similar immunological features to human T lymphotropic virus-type 1-associated myelopathy/tropical spastic paraparesis. Clin Exp Immunol 2009;156:455–62.

71. Tschachler E, Franchini G. Infective dermatitis: a pabulum for human T-lymphotrophic virus type I leukemogenesis? Arch Dermatol 1998; 134:487–8.

72. De Oliveira MD, Vieira MD, Primo J, et al. Flower cells in patients with infective dermatitis associated with HTLV-1. J Clin Virol 2010;48(4): 288–90.

73. Bittencourt AL, Oliveira MD, Argolo J, et al. Infective dermatitis associated with human-T-cell lymphotropic virus type-1 is a pre-ATL condition? In Annals of the 22nd European Academy of

Dermatology & Venereology Congress. Istanbul (Turkey), October 2–6, 2013.

74. Imaizumi Y, Iwanaga M, Tsukasaki K, et al. Natural course of HTLV-1 carriers with monoclonal proliferation of T lymphocytes ("pre-ATL") in a 20-year follow-up study. Blood 2005;105(2):903–4.

75. De The G, Bomford R. An HTLV-I vaccine: why, how, for whom? AIDS Res Hum Retroviruses 1993;9:381–6.

76. Manns A, Hisada M, La Grenade L. Human T-lymphotropic virus type I infection. Lancet 1999;353: 1951–8.

Index

Note: Page numbers of article titles are in **boldface** type.

A

Acid peels
    and keloids, hypertrophic scars, and striae, 199
Acne keloidalis nuchae. See *Folliculitis keloidalis nuchae.*
Acquired immunodeficiency syndrome. See *Human immunodeficiency virus.*
AD. See *Atopic dermatitis.*
Adult T-cell leukemia/lymphoma
    and human T-cell lymphotropic virus type 1, 237–239, 242–245
Advances and challenges in hair restoration of curly afrocentric hair, **163–171**
African ancestry
    and eumelanin, 114, 116, 117
    and hair texture, 113–119
    and integumentary phenotypes, 113–119
    and melanocortin 1 receptor, 114, 117
    and pigmentation, 113–119
    and pigmentation and hair texture, 113–119
    and thermoregulation, 117, 118
    and ultraviolet radiation, 114–118
    and vitamin D deficiency, 117, 118
Afro-textured hair disorders
    and alopecia areata, 147, 153–160
    and alopecia due to hair breakage, 147
    and androgenetic alopecia, 147
    and biopsy, 150
    and central centrifugal cicatricial alopecia, 148
    and dermatoscopy, 145–150
    and discoid lupus erythematosus, 148, 149
    and dissecting cellulitis of the scalp, 149
    and frontal fibrosing alopecia, 149
    and lichen planopilaris, 149
    and normal scalp, 145, 146
    and pili annulati, 149, 150
    and tinea capitis, 146, 147
    and traction alopecia, 148
Afrocentric hair
    and hair restoration, 163–170
Alopecia areata
    and afro-textured hair disorders, 147
Androgenetic alopecia
    and afro-textured hair disorders, 147
Antioxidants
    and cosmeceuticals, 141
ATLL. See *Adult T-cell leukemia/lymphoma.*
Atopic dermatitis

and human T-cell lymphotropic virus type 1, 240–244
Automated devices
    for hair restoration, 170

B

Bacillary angiomatosis
    and HIV-associated dermatoses, 213
Bacterial infections
    and HIV-associated dermatoses, 213–215
Barrier function
    and cosmeceuticals, 140

C

CADR. See *Cutaneous adverse drug reactions.*
CCCA. See *Central centrifugal cicatricial alopecia.*
Central centrifugal cicatricial alopecia
    and afro-textured hair disorders, 148
    causes of, 178, 179
    and chronic inflammation, 178, 179
    clinical features of, 176, 177
    epidemiology of, 177, 178
    and family history, 179
    and female pattern hair loss, 178
    and follicular degeneration syndrome, 175–177
    and hair care practices, 174, 178
    and hair cleansing, 174
    and hair morphology, 173, 174
    and hair restoration, 164–166, 168, 169
    and hair straightening, 174
    and hair styling, 174
    histopathology of, 177
    history of, 175, 176
    and hot combing, 174–176, 178
    and microorganisms, 178, 179
    and scarring hair loss, 175–179
    treatment of, 179
Central centrifugal cicatricial alopecia: what has been achieved, current clues for future research, **173–181**
Clinical presentations of severe cutaneous drug reactions in HIV-infected Africans, **227–235**
Cosmeceuticals
    and antioxidants, 141
    and barrier function, 140
    claims of, 139, 140
    development of, 139

Dermatol Clin 32 (2014) 249–254
http://dx.doi.org/10.1016/S0733-8635(14)00010-2
0733-8635/14/$ – see front matter © 2014 Elsevier Inc. All rights reserved

Moving?

Make sure your subscription moves with you!

To notify us of your new address, find your **Clinics Account Number** (located on your mailing label above your name), and contact customer service at:

Email: journalscustomerservice-usa@elsevier.com

800-654-2452 (subscribers in the U.S. & Canada)
314-447-8871 (subscribers outside of the U.S. & Canada)

Fax number: 314-447-8029

Elsevier Health Sciences Division
Subscription Customer Service
3251 Riverport Lane
Maryland Heights, MO 63043

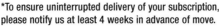
*To ensure uninterrupted delivery of your subscription, please notify us at least 4 weeks in advance of move.

Printed and bound by CPI Group (UK) Ltd, Croydon, CR0 4YY

03/10/2024

01040374-0008